THE MIND AS HEALER
The New Heresy

THE MIND AS HEALER

The New Heresy

Edited by
Onslow H. Wilson, Ph.D.

Transcription of addresses given at the First Annual Metaphysiology Symposium, focusing on The Mind as Healer. Held at the Egyptian Museum, San Jose, California on September 27, 1986 and at the Pasadena City College on April 18, 1987.

Published by
INSIGHTS AND SOURCES CORPORATION
Plainfield, Indiana — Fremont, California

International Standard Book Number
ISBN O-943325-00-5

Library of Congress Catalog Card Number: 87-80443

Authors' Names: Dr. Willis Harman, Dr. Kenneth Pelletier,
Dr. Martin Rossman, Dr. Alan Brauer, Dr. Onslow H.
Wilson, Brendan O'Regan, Marilyn Ferguson and Dr. Ray
Gottlieb

Title of Book: *The Mind as Healer — The New Heresy*

Edition: First

Date of Publication: June, 1987

Publisher: Insights and Sources Corporation, P.O. Box 1858,
Fremont, California 94538

Publication Number: 51E00187

Graphics By Jerry Chapman

TABLE OF CONTENTS

FOREWORD

INSIGHTS AND SOURCES CORPORATION is particularly pleased to publish the proceedings of the Metaphysiology Symposiums since they simultaneously address two diverse but pertinent issues of great interest at this time.

The first of these issues concerns the use of one's own mind for the promotion of one's personal health.

The second concerns the gathering momentum for a science expanded by new tools and directions hitherto regarded as "off limits."

Interest in self-healing has grown along with a strong undercurrent of discontent with the health delivery system at the very time that modern medicine is dazzling us with new techniques and instrumentation. Many people are coming to the view that they should more directly involve their "inner physician," with the licensed practitioner filling the role of consultant. This inward, rather than outward, view of one's health has revealed to many that they have therapeutic capabilities of surprising efficacy. Fortunately, as this publication shows, there are experienced practitioners who share the view that the individual patient has within himself or herself seemingly unlimited therapeutic possibilities. Our minds can not only produce psychosomatic illness, they can produce psychosomatic therapy. This casting aside of imagined restrictions of the mind is opening new and exciting vistas of potential knowledge.

If our about-to-be-discovered new knowledge were where we expected it to be, in all likelihood we would have discovered it already. It remains hidden from us simply because it lies where we have not as yet looked, perhaps because we assume, **BEFORE INVESTIGATION**, that the area is unfruitful, does not lend itself to our instrumentation, or is subject to ridicule.

This leads to the second issue discussed in the Symposiums; the expansion of science into areas regarded as "off limits." From the time of Francis Bacon, who insisted on the close and methodical observation of the facts (after dismissal of prejudices and preconceptions of all kinds), until now, there has been little doubt that science has developed many wonders and expanded capabilities to almost unimaginable breath. However, at this stage of our inquiries, it is becoming more and more apparent to thinking people that expanded tools of investigation must be utilized to probe areas that have been avoided, or found resistant to the quantitative, sequential approach at which modern science excels.

This publication has a great deal to say about this new view which Willis Harman, in the introduction, calls "**THE NEW HERESY.**"

Are we now at another epochal transition that will see profuse flowing of new knowledge and insights into a changed reality? Reading the addresses of The Metaphysiology Symposiums certainly makes it seem likely.

Currently we are hampered by two views of the mind's abilities.

First, we reject out of hand hypotheses regarding the mind's potential because we cannot reasonably imagine such capabilities. Indeed, there is much evidence that the mind's limitations are largely unknown, hence the most fruitful investigative mode is to assume no limitations. This publication pursues this very point with fascinating practical results.

Second, incidents of strange phenomena are considered hoaxes unless they can be regularly replicated. Yet, lack of replication does not prevent general acceptance of many of the principles of astronomy. That a given phenomenon is very rare and cannot be replicated at will is often not as important as the fact that it occurred at all. And if it did occur, should we not find ways to increase its incidence and thus increase our knowledge? This very approach was taken at CERN (the European high energy physics research center in Geneva, Switzerland) with the discovery, in 1983, of the W^+, W^-, and Z^0 particles operating within the atomic nucleus. An examination of millions of events was made to search for the exceedingly rare four or five that revealed the weak force bosons that implement radiation. This search for a most-difficult-to-replicate event was worthy of a Nobel Prize.

Should we do less where the mind and consciousness are concerned? As this publication reveals, there are those with expert training who are willing to take the same approach in dealing with the mind and health.

In transcribing these addresses we have tried to preserve the flavor of an oral presentation so as to convey the enthusiasm that was generated at the symposiums. As one who attended the symposiums and felt this enthusiasm in the presentations, my hope is that this publication will bring the same excitement to its readers.

Readers who are not scientists or physicians themselves will appreciate that these are not hard to read scientific papers prepared for publication in a scientific format but represent the informal sharing of ideas.

Our special thanks to Mary Jessie Cisneroz, Rosemary E. P. Church, Kathleen Lee and Michael Kent for their transcribing, editing and proofreading.

Marshall Kent, President, INSIGHTS AND SOURCES CORPORATION

INTRODUCTION

The Current Crisis in Science:
The Outlook for an Extended Methodology
and Content

By Willis Harman

Editor's note: *The scientific revolution of the seventeenth century shaped every aspect of the modern world. It was, in essence, a* **heresy**—*a widening group of people who first whispered, and later said aloud, "Reality is not the way the religious authorities told us!" A new authority system replaced the old—the authority system we call* **empirical science**, *and that changed everything.*

In the late twentieth century a **new heresy** *is abroad: a widening group of persons are observing, "Reality is not the way the secular authorities told us either!" Empirical science is misleading in its description of the world. This new heresy, like the "scientific heresy" before it, will change everything. Because it proposes a different set of assumptions about reality than those which underlie the modern world, the trans-modern world of the 21st century will be as different from modern times as those are from the Middle Ages.*

In this introduction to **The Mind As Healer — The New Heresy,** *Willis Harman explores this challenging possibility.*

Science as it stands would appear to be beset with serious problems. Attempts to deal with the full nature of living organisms have led some scientists to propose something like vitalism; this has been sharply criticized by others. Attempts to create an adequate science of human experience have led some to introduce, in Roger Sperry's phrase, "inner conscious awareness as a causal reality"; to others this concept seems to violate a basic deterministic assumption inherent in the very idea of science. For thousands of years there have been persistent reports of the inner discovery of a basic spiritual nature; yet to many, science is supposed to have discarded such prescientific superstitions long ago. Thrusts in a more holistic direction like "deep ecology" and "transpersonal psychology" are hailed by some and deplored by others.

One wonders if we have not become trapped in the quagmire of our own dogmas. Is there not a way to escape from these dilemmas without sacrificing any of the intellectual rigor, open spirit of inquiry, and public validation of knowledge that characterize science at its best?

In exploring that question I would like to start with the puzzle that has seemed most perplexing—namely, what to do about the key aspects of conscious experience, particularly comprehension, volition, intention, attention, and freedom of will. After all, the only experience of reality that we have *directly* is our own conscious awareness. There could be no science without a phenomenon of *comprehension*. Our experience of ourselves and our environment is modulated by what we decide to pay *attention* to. The experience of *volition* is too real for us to accept easily that free will is merely "A prescientific concept describing behavior for which we have not yet found a cause" (as B. F. Skinner once put it). Yet we have been making do with a science which was intrinsically incapable of dealing with such concepts.

THE PROBLEM OF CONSCIOUSNESS

It was the hallmark of the behavioral science's emphasis of the 1950s that only what was ultimately measurable could be the subject of scientific inquiry. Thus consciousness, in scientific terms, was reduced to behavior (e.g. apparent awareness, responsiveness) and neurophysiological phenomena (e.g. brain waves), observable from outside the organism. Early approaches to dealing with inner conscious awareness in its own terms (i.e. introspectionism and phenomenology) had been discredited. Rigorously inclined behavioral scientists insisted that it would be impossible to construct a reliable science based on self-reports of inner, subjective experience.

This behavioral predilection became quite strong, particularly in the United States. Nevertheless, there remained the sneaking suspicion on the part of many, scientists as well as nonscientists, that science had a hidden bias: something important was being left out.

It was in the area of exceptional abilities that it became most clear that all was not well with our scientific methodology. Down through the centuries a variety of anomalous phenomena, including clairvoyant remote viewing, telepathic communication, levitation and teleportation, "instantaneous" spiritual healing, and other so-called psychic phenomena, have been reported. Explanations of fraud, collusion, error, and self-deception have been offered, and refuted, as to why these reports are probably mistaken. Famous and competent scientists have arrayed themselves on both sides of the debate. A half-century ago it seemed fairly clear that in spite of the unwavering claims of a few persons doing research in the dubious field of parapsychology, the better educated and more sophisticated public felt confident that scientific advance was making the genuineness of the phenomena decreasingly plausible. In more recent years, however, the Parapsychology Association has been admitted to the roster of the

American Association for the Advancement of Science, and there are clear indications from an assortment of kinds of evidence that the more highly educated portion of the public are finding the existence of such phenomena more plausible.

This state of affairs is, to say the least, puzzling. Why is belief in the existence and significance of these phenomena so persistent in spite of the admittedly inconclusive nature of the scientific research findings? And why, if these are genuine phenomena, do we not know more about them by now?

Part of the answer was given by Nobel laureate Roger Sperry in a salient paper entitled "Changing Priorities" (*1981 Annual Review of Neurosciences*), where he said:

> Current concepts of the mind-brain relation involve a direct break with the long-established materialist and behaviorist doctrine that has dominated neuroscience for many decades. Instead of renouncing or ignoring consciousness, the new interpretation gives full recognition to the primacy of inner conscious awareness as a causal reality.

"Inner conscious awareness as a causal reality" was expressly denied by the positivistic bias of an older science. Thus a key factor in the puzzle is the fact that *accepted scientific methodology is not well adapted to investigation of phenomena where "consciousness as a causal reality" appears to be a central factor.*

THE BIAS OF WESTERN SCIENCE

The observation that Western science is characterized by a certain bias should not be either surprising nor appear as a criticism. For one thing, there is inevitably a partiality in the support pattern. Modern society's institutions tend to give preferential support to research that appears likely to benefit the economy or to bring advances in military or medical technology. In the early stages of science much of the impetus came from the needs of military engineering and celestial navigation.

Another kind of bias arises because of the methodological difficulties in some areas. It was reasonable enough, in the early years of empirical science, to concentrate efforts where the conduct of inquiry seemed a little more straightforward—in mechanics and anatomy, for example, as compared with explorations of the human mind.

There was furthermore, in those early years, a tacit agreement with the Church that the upstart scientific enterprise would not stray too far into the territory of the soul and spirit, since those were the province of ecclesiastical rather than empirical authority.

Thus for practical and political reasons that were quite valid at the time, the scientific enterprise early became characterized by three assumptions which we shall list and discuss briefly. They were:

> 1. The *objectivist* assumption, that there is an objective universe which can be explored by the methods of scientific inquiry, and which can be approximated, progressively more precisely, by quantitative models;
> 2. The *positivist* assumption, that what is scientifically "real" must take as its basic data only that which is physically observable; and
> 3. The *reductionist* assumption, that scientific explanation consists in explaining complex phenomena in terms of more elemental events (e.g. gas temperature and pressure in terms of the motions of the molecules; human behavior in terms of stimulus and response).

These characteristics have seemed so integral to the scientific method that it is hard to imagine they would ever be displaced. Yet the data of exceptional abilities challenge them in a way that may bring about a major revolutionary advance. (Indeed, Michael Polanyi, in his keen analysis of scientific method, *Personal Knowledge,* argues that the fundamental premises of science are continually undergoing change: They are never quite the same after a scientific discovery is made as they were before.)

The nature of these methodological challenges is seen most clearly through examination of three topics: (a) the need for holistic models; (b) the influence of unconscious mental processes; and (c) the role of the observer.

HOLISTIC MODELS AND HIERARCHICAL CAUSES

It may seem almost obvious that *the whole is qualitatively different from the sum of the parts.* A chemical compound displays qualities quite different from the qualities of any of its separate ingredients. An ecological system has characteristics one would not have suspected from simply examining its component organisms. A culture has characteristics that are not simply the sum of the behaviors of the individuals who compose it. The human body is not simply the sum of the organs and tissues that compose it.

Yet that basic principle has implications with regard to causative models which have not been appreciated through the history of science; that lack of appreciation has led to bitter dissents. *If characteristics emerge at higher system levels that are qualitatively different from those at lower levels, then the sciences appropriate to different levels will be qualitatively different.* The science of cells is qualitatively different from the science of organisms, which in turn differs from the science of ecological systems.

A simple extension of this principle leads to the concept of a hierarchy of complementary and mutually non-contradictory "explanations" for the same phenomenon. The factors that enter into an explanation at one level of system complexity may be meaningless at another level. Thus at one level of system hierarchy a conscious decision to act may be part of the explanation, whereas at another level we can comprehend only non-volitional, physical forces.

For example, suppose that I come down with a cold. At one level of explanation we may say that a virus "causes" the cold. But viruses, bacteria and a vast assortment of other microorganisms inhabit the space known as "my body" all the time. If we add in the body cells, I am "really" a vast ecological community of microorganisms which exist in a state of largely cooperative balance—most of the time. If this ecology gets out of balance, perhaps following my taking a chill, then I am said to have a particular disease, characterized by that imbalance. Put another way, the body's immune system functioning—which, after all, is the consequence of actions of a host of "friendly" microorganisms, T cells and the like—is impaired, and that is why I have the cold. That is another level of explanation.

At yet another explanatory level we may observe that the reason the ecology of bodily microorganisms got out of balance was something called "stress." Stress is a psychological response to the environment such that various glandular secretions increase, and the body gets ready for "fight or flight." Repeated or continuous stress in situations where fleeing is unseemly and physical fighting is impermissible can lead to malfunction of the immune system—hence susceptibility to colds.

These three explanations, all valid in their own way, are at different levels in some sort of hierarchy. Moving from the first to the second to the third, there is a progressive increase in the amount of the universe included in the system under consideration. Furthermore, the causal agents are different at the different levels. At one level it may be the cold virus; at another, the condition of the body's immune system; at another, attitudes toward home and work which bring on the stress condition. These causal agents are progressively less physical and more abstract. Note that the abstract causes are not less "scientific" than the others; they merely occur at different levels in the hierarchy.

At a less sophisticated stage of science there was a tendency to consider the level of physical causation to be somehow more "real" than the more abstract levels (positivism). Thus for example, there was considerable initial resistance to the idea of psychosomatic illness, or the idea that positive emotions might have a salutary effect on the body's immune system. Furthermore, "scientific explanation" tended to imply interpretation at the level of physical causation (reductionism). Thus teleological causes (i.e. explanations involving purpose) were ruled out. A reaction of the arm to an external stimulus could be dealt with scientifically, but an arm movement *for the purpose of reaching a desired object* could not. The need is increasingly apparent to somehow extend science beyond the restrictions of this predilection for the physical level.

BEING CONSCIOUS OF THE UNCONSCIOUS

Starting with the early researchers into hypnosis, including Freud, we find increasing acceptance of some concept of unconscious mental processes. At this point, few findings in the social sciences are as well established as the discovery (or perhaps more accurately, the rediscovery) that the greater portion of our mental activity goes on outside of conscious awareness. We believe, value, choose, and know unconsciously as well as consciously. Yet we typically live, think and behave without taking seriously the implications of that fact.

The way we perceive reality is strongly influenced by unconsciously held beliefs. The phenomena of denial and resistance in psychotherapy illustrate how thoroughly one tends not to see things that would be threatening to deeply held images or are in conflict with deeply held beliefs. Research on hypnosis, self- and experimenter-expectations, authoritarianism and prejudice, subliminal perception, and selective attention has demonstrated over and over that our perceptions and "reality checks" are influenced far more than is ordinarily assumed by beliefs, attitudes, and other mental processes of which a large portion is unconscious.

The phenomena of hypnosis, in particular, emphasize dramatically how changes in unconscious beliefs, brought about in this case by suggestion, can alter perception and experience. Through hypnotic suggestion one can be led to perceive what isn't there, or fail to perceive what is there, or experience limits that aren't real, or transcend limits thought to be real.

Enculturation is not in essence different from hypnosis. Through repeated and persistent suggestion, especially in infancy when there is a high degree of openness, each one of us is inevitably *culturally hypnotized* to perceive the world in the way our own culture perceives it. We find it curious that other "primitive" or "traditional" cultures should perceive reality in the ways they do—so obviously discrepant with the modern scientific world view. It is much harder to entertain the thought that we in modern Western society might have our own cultural peculiarities in the form of limits and distortions. Since Western science is the most effective knowledge system ever devised (for achieving the goals of Western society), it seems reasonable to consider our culture superior, our values "normal," our predilections "natural," and our perceived world "real."

Thus it has been especially humbling—and to some, shocking—to come to realize that Western science, like the knowledge system of every other society, is parochial to our society. The findings of scientific research continually bring us to reshape our picture of reality, to be sure. But *the nature of that scientific inquiry is in turn shaped by the culture within which it developed.*

The recognition has not come easily that despite the unquestioned prowess of the West's scientific capabilities, there might be a subtle but pervasive and momentous bias in its emphasis on *pragmatically useful knowledge,* and on *manipulative rationality.*

As cultural anthropologists have discovered over and over (and as noted above), people who grow up in different societies develop differing pictures of reality. In those different pictures, there are differences in what is considered "useful." For many centuries the various cultures of the Indian subcontinent, for example, have placed great stress on knowledge that related to inner understanding, psychological knowledge in the broadest sense. Ancient Chinese civilization, on the other hand, placed special emphasis on knowledge pertaining to social relationships—to manners, ethics, deportment, social solidarity. Despite the demonstrated Chinese ingenuity, exemplified by their early invention of gunpowder, rockets, paper, printing, etc., they lacked the interest in exploiting technological knowledge that later characterized the West. A primary question for them was: How, through culture, may humankind become one; coherent, peaceful, and creative?

The prevailing values of Western society after the Middle Ages placed great value on the manipulation of the physical environment through technology; scientific knowledge eventually, after the mid-nineteenth century, came increasingly to serve technology. That knowledge was perceived as useful which led to further technology—that is, knowledge contributing to the ability to *predict and control.* With this emphasis on prediction- and control-focused knowledge the world gradually came to be perceived as subject to that kind of understanding and manipulation; experience that might contradict such a positivist picture was unconsciously screened out.

Thus we confront a bit of a paradox. The scientific knowledge that has been gathered about unconscious mental processes has alerted us to a bias in that very science. Furthermore, it becomes clear that in dealing with an area like exceptional abilities, the effects of unconscious processes comprise essential aspects of the phenomena.

THE INFLUENCE OF THE OBSERVER

Every student of college physics knows that the act of observation disturbs the phenomenon being studied; it is impossible to separate the observer from the observed. Every psychotherapist and anthropologist knows that one cannot truly view another individual or another culture without to some degree perturbing that which is being studied. Yet scientists are understandably reluctant to give up the ideal of scientific *objectivity,* with its close relationship to that prime characteristic of scientific findings, *reliability.*

Consider the commonplace testing of the efficacy of a new analgesic by giving the drug to a large population of subjects and making a statistical analysis of the data. In judging the merits of such research there would tend to be a shared understanding that pain is a subjective response affected by all sorts of subtle variables, such as the subject's desire to cooperate with the experimenter, placebo effect, deliberate or inadvertent suppression of pain by autosuggestion, individual uniqueness, variability of the subject's responses from day to day, etc. Even with all the sophistication of double-blind techniques one would not expect, in research that so centrally involves self-reports of subjectively felt pain, to be able to apply rigid definitions of "objectivity" and "replicability." Yet we are not inclined to be hypercritical of the results of such research just because of this impossibility of demonstrating strict objectivity and replicability.

In other research more directly related to exploring the powers of mind, the problems with objectivity and replicability become more acute. Take for example the reported remission of symptoms of cancer, AIDS, etc. through systematic use of inner imagery and autosuggestion. Careful work has been carried out by competent researchers, and the results strongly suggest the existence of a genuine phenomenon. Yet because of the absence of some concept of a "mechanism" to account for the phenomenon, research findings purporting to demonstrate it are expected to meet especially stringent requirements. By these strict standards, they fail to pass the test. Researchers with positive beliefs about the phenomena tend to get positive results, and skeptics tend to get negative results. And the results are erratic even under what appear to be similar conditions; we seem to have here a sporadic rather than a repeatable phenomenon.

The skeptical interpret these characteristics of the research as evidence of the nonexistence of the phenomena. However, they can also be interpreted as indications of inappropriate demands for "objectivity" and "replicability." As is well known, human beings make choices at unconscious as well as conscious levels (e.g. addiction—an unconscious choice overruling a conscious one; or guilt feelings—a disapproving message from some part of the unconscious mind regarding a choice made consciously). But in self-healing of cancer, unconscious as well as conscious choices are involved; the person may want one thing at one level of the mind and something else at another. With this uncontrollable factor entering in, strict replicability is impossible. Furthermore, if one postulates the possibility of minds interacting at a distance—which research on the "anomalies" or "psychic phenomena" strongly suggests—then it becomes apparent that the conscious and unconscious state of mind of the experimenter can affect the healing of the subject, so strict objectivity is an impossibility.

Morris Berman, in *The Reenchantment of the World*, argues with particular trenchancy that an adequate science cannot be based on attempting to know Nature from the outside, through controlled experiments in which phenomena are examined in abstraction from their context. In extended science, we understand that Nature is revealed only in our relations with it, and phenomena can be known only in context (that is, through participant observation).

THE DEEPER IMPORTANCE OF THE CONSCIOUSNESS ISSUE

The critical importance of this issue of "consciousness as causal reality" is emphasized by further remarks of Sperry:

> Beliefs concerning the ultimate purpose and meaning of life and the accompanying worldview perspectives that mold beliefs of right and wrong are critically dependent, directly or by implication, on concepts regarding the conscious self and the mind-brain relation and the kinds of life goals and cosmic views which these allow. Directly or indirectly social values depend . . . on whether consciousness is believed to be mortal, immortal, reincarnate, or cosmic . . . localized and brainbound or essentially universal. . . . Recent conceptual developments in the mind-brain sciences rejecting reductionism and materialistic determinism on the one hand, and dualism on the other, clear the way for a rational approach to the theory and prescription of values and to a natural fusion of science and religion.

Thus the Western scientific neglect of inner experience has directly contributed to our present confusion about values. For it is ultimately in this realm of the subjective, the transcendent, and the spiritual, that all individuals and all societies have found the basis for their deepest value commitments and sense of meaning.

But how to deal with the subjective in a way that is true to the spirit of scientific inquiry, and yet not in the process so distort it that in the end the resulting science is no longer true to its subject? That is the puzzling question. It has a long history.

Throughout the ages, individuals and communities seem repeatedly to have come upon the awe-inspiring creative factors and forces of the human psyche. Time and again, as an outcome of such discoveries, great philosophies and religions have come into being, which for a while profoundly influenced the course of human events. But time and again, also, the knowledge appears to have been lost or become inaccessible, or at best preserved within small, closed esoteric groups. With the vogue of positivistic science in the earlier part of this century, the religious meanings associated with such experiences were rather thoroughly debunked, and serious exploration of the creative unconscious was discouraged.

Recently, however, there has been a resurgence of interest—both in the broader society (in various meditative disciplines, mind-body approaches to health care, arcane studies and religious philosophies) and also in the scientific community, in research on consciousness. Scientists of considerable stature such as neuroscientist Roger Sperry, physicist David Bohm, neurophysiologist Sir John Eccles, and biologist Rupert Sheldrake have argued what would have been rank heresy only a decade or so ago, namely that there are unmeasurable, nonphysical aspects to reality that have to be taken into account scientifically because they are part of human experience—not the experience of the physical senses, but the experience of the deep intuition and of alternative states of consciousness. As William James had written, "No account of the universe in its totality can be final which leaves these data disregarded."

The question which troubled scientists a half century ago, "Does mind exist?" (since it cannot be measured) seems strangely anachronistic today. The question remains, however, how to study mind in a way compatible with the scientific tradition of open inquiry and public validation of knowledge, and yet not be bound by too narrow and inappropriate a concept of "scientific method."

A CRISIS OF SCIENCE

It has been apparent for some time that modern science is experiencing a crisis. In the introductory paragraph to his *A Sense of the Cosmos*, theologian Jacob Needleman wrote in 1975:

> Once the hope of mankind, modern science has now become the object of such mistrust and disappointment that it will probably never again speak with its old authority. The crisis of ecology, the threat of atomic war, and the disruption of the patterns of human life by advanced technology have all eroded what was once a general trust in the *goodness* of science. And the appearance in our society of alien metaphysical systems, of "new religions" sourced in the East, and of ideas and fragments of teachings emanating from ancient times have all contributed doubt about the *truth* of science. Even among scientists themselves there are signs of a metaphysical rebellion. Modern man is searching for a new world view.

As with the crises of life, we may be reasonably sure that this crisis is but a phase preparatory to an evolutionary advance. The dilemma is especially apparent in the area of exceptional abilities, defined broadly as above. To summarize, it is this: The enterprise of modern science very early became identified with the three assumptions of objectivism, positivism, and reductionism. It then experienced great difficulty in dealing with many phenomena and aspects of human life. These include, for example, such everyday phenomena as attention, volition, comprehension, and the exquisite regulation of the physical organism; the extraordinary, "paranormal" phenomena that seem to intrude from time to time; the unconscious processing of information associated with intuitive insight and creative inspiration; the profound inner experiences that lead to the deepest value commitments of individuals and societies; and the whole realm of spiritual and religious experience, which one can hardly write off in its entirety (although some zealous philosophers of science have tried to do so).

Science has a long history of defending the bulwarks against the persistent reports of phenomena and experiences that "don't fit in." *Suppose, instead, we take the opposite approach; namely, to assume the validity of any type of human experience or extraordinary ability which is consistently reported down through the ages, or across cultures, and explore the characteristics of a science that could accommodate these.*

TOWARD A MORE COMPREHENSIVE SCIENCE

We have seen in the above discussion that such a more comprehensive science will have to include some concept of hierarchical models. (Among the foremost contributors to the idea of hierarchical models in science are G.N.M. Tyrrell, in *Grades of Significance,* Michael Polanyi in *Personal Knowledge,* and Arthur Koestler in the proceedings of the 1965 Alpach Symposium on "Beyond Reductionism".)

One such fourfold schema of explanatory levels is suggested here. One level is that of the present physical sciences. Another level, equally valid in a scientific sense and clearly necessary in the biological and health sciences, is one characterized by holistic concepts like "organism" and teleological concepts like "function." A third level admits of even more holistic and abstract concepts like "personal health" and "personality" and "individual purpose." A fourth level, required if the deep subjective experience of untold mystics, prophets, artists, and poets, down through the ages, is to be honored, is the suprapersonal, which would include such a concept as "universal purpose". This is shown in the diagram below.

Four Levels of Models and Explanations

Level	Health Example	Evolution Example
4. Suprapersonal	Spiritual health; wholeness	Universal purpose
3. Personal	Individual biological health	Individual purpose
2. Organism	Organ function; illness	System function; natural selection
1. Physical	Metabolism rate; body temperature	Molecular biology; mutation; physical characteristics

It is apparent that an extensive "level-1" science already exists. In the life sciences and psychiatric theory there are fragments of a "level-2" science which repudiates the claims of some molecular biologists that eventually all behavior is explained by the genes. As for "level-3" science, humanistic psychology and sociology are even more fragmentary. At the fourth level we find attempts such as transpersonal psychology and Tibetan Buddhist psychology. James Lovelock's "Gaia Hypothesis" considers the Earth as a self-regulating organism; in its most widely accepted form it is a level-2 concept, but some would attribute consciousness to the planet in a level-4 hypothesis. At level-4 there is the problem of a limited number of qualified observers (qualified in terms of their own inner development) and it has been extremely difficult to avoid the pitfalls of dogma and cult.

A number of features of such a multileveled science need to be noted.

MODELS AND METAPHORS. It is apparent that the models and metaphors used at one explanatory level may be obviously inappropriate at another. The holistic metaphors appropriate to considering human personality are "nonphysical" and do not appear at the physical level; on the other hand, atomistic explanations of organic processes at the physical level leave out the essence of what is being studied at the higher levels.

Perhaps the first thing to be noted is that there need be no claim to exclusivity in terms of which level is ultimately "real." Physicists led the way in the recognition that reality is too rich to be fully expressed in any model, theory, metaphor, or equation. Wave models do not invalidate particle models, and vice-versa; the two metaphors are *complementary* not contradictory.

A scientist may behave professionally as though the physical level describes what is "real." Another scientist (or for that matter, the same one) may lead his/her personal life as though only the suprapersonal level of mind and spirit points to the ultimately real. There is no contradiction involved, and the individual does not become a schizoid personality for holding both views at the same time. Indeed, a person may be a better scientist for not having to fight so strongly to defend the positivism and reductionism appropriate to the physical level.

There are aberrations to be avoided, arising from adopting too extreme a position. The extreme positivist, reductionist position leads to having to deny the reality of the most immediate experience, such as that of attention and volition. The extreme suprapersonal position can result in a person who is ineffective through not being "grounded."

REFRAMING OF UNFRUITFUL CONTROVERSY. Many of the scientific controversies of the past disappear when we reframe them in terms of levels of explanations. The behaviorist issue is clearly a matter of a certain group of scientists insisting that they will not deal with what is not at the level of physical measurability. The vitalism controversy, to take another example, becomes a matter of recognizing that when dealing with living systems higher explanatory levels are required than when dealing with most inorganic phenomena. Dualistic approaches amount to considering only two levels, rather than at least four. Miraculous healings, such as those meeting the stringent criteria set by the International Medical Commission at Lourdes, in France, may in the end be considered to fit at the suprapersonal level and to not contravene the usefulness of the physical and organismic levels of explanation for many other purposes.

One such perennial controversy has been over interpretation of the phenomena of *morphogenesis*. Morphogenesis, literally the birth of form, is particularly evident in healing, regeneration (restoration of a mutilated organism), and embryonic growth. An extreme form of regeneration is found in some simple animals, like hydra or planaria, where a tiny fragment of the organism can regenerate a complete individual. In embryonic growth, multiplication of a single cell eventually results in the formation of a complete organism, with many diverse cells performing widely differentiated functions. In order to explain the phenomena, the concept has been introduced of a vital force, peculiar to living organisms, that directs form and development. "Vitalism," as this idea has been termed, has in general been very controversial in the scientific community. The term "morphogenetic field" has been used since the 1920s to describe the organizing principle whereby the many cells are guided to combine, with differentiated functions, to produce a living organism of particular form. (The same term was later extended by Rupert Sheldrake to account for complex instinctual behaviors in animals.) But there seems to be no satisfactory way of explaining morphogenesis at the physical level; some higher-level concept appears to be required.

A somewhat similar controversy is present with regard to evolution (complicated by the fact that Fundamentalist Christianity is also in the act). The prevailing neo-Darwinist theory tends to account for the evolution of high-order species through random mutation and natural selection. This, however, leaves many puzzles, not the least of which is that posed by structures (such as the two eyes for binocular vision) which would appear to have no survival value in any intermediate stage, so that it is hard to imagine their evolution taking place in any sort of incremental way—and equally hard to imagine through a sudden transformational leap. It seems possible that a more adequate theory of the evolutionary process will eventually include both the neo-Darwinist sort of mechanism and some higher-level morphogenetic directing force, something like a universal (or at least planetary) mind.

Not all such controversy is easily removed. For example, astrology has been sustained for thousands of years by empirical generalizations based on the predictions of horoscopes; if there is ever to be a robust theory of astrological influence it will obviously have to be at a suprapersonal level. Again, the 17th century destruction of belief in phenomena related to witchcraft, shamanism, animism, etc. was in the face of overwhelming evidence supporting existence of the phenomena; new kinds of acceptable explanations may well appear in time, but they will have to be at a personal (e.g. as phenomena of hypnosis) or suprapersonal level.

Particular mention should be made of the principle of parsimony—the idea that a simpler and more aesthetically elegant conceptualization should be preferred to a more elaborate or complex one, when both accommodate the known facts. This principle would seem to have been often misapplied in the past, when it has been used to disallow explanations at the higher levels in favor of straining to reinterpret (or disallow) data to fit the explanation into the physical level.

Explanatory concepts at one level may be very useful in complementing the primary explanations of phenomena at some different level. The conceptualizations at the physical level, for example, may add rich detail to psychosomatic processes where the basic explanation appears to be at a higher level. The highly sophisticated suprapersonal conceptualizations of the Tibetan Buddhist psychologies, on the other hand, may contribute important insights into processes at the personal and organismic levels.

QUESTIONS ASKED. Questions not appropriate at one level of models may nevertheless fit at another. Thus teleological questions have no place in the level of reductionistic science of physical reality. At the next level, however, it is appropriate to ask about the function of the body's immune system, or of elaborate instinctive patterns in animal behavior. At the next level volition may be acceptable as a causal factor, and personality is a meaningful construct. At the suprapersonal level questions about "other kinds of consciousness" achieved in meditative states, and guidance of choices by some kind of deep intuition, may be meaningful.

In the past, scientists have tended to insist that teleological questions and value-focused questions are not appropriate to science. Of course, they have always been asked in some areas, such as the health sciences. A question about the function of some part of the body's regulatory system is teleological, and certainly a question about what leads toward health is value-focused.

To those who still ask whether these kinds of questions are appropriate to science, one can reply with the question, "If not science, then who?" There is no other authority in modern society with the prestige of science to ask these important questions.

DATA ADMITTED. It seems clear that the new science will in some way have to deal with subjective reports of deep inner experience. When this has been put forward in the past (e.g. in introspectionism, phenomenology, gestalt psychology) the idea was rejected by the main body of scientists. Perhaps it will come forward now in more sophisticated form.

At the level of "physical reality" admissible data is primarily in the form of quantifiable physical observation. At the organism level somewhat more holistic kinds of observations become important, such as instinctive behavior patterns, or the functioning of the digestive system. Self-reports of inner, subjective experience become relevant at the personal level, and essentially comprise the sole source of data at the suprapersonal level.

THEORIES CONSIDERED. Reductionism has been so characteristic of most science that one almost automatically thinks of scientific explanation in those terms. We understand (scientifically) a phenomenon when we can describe it in terms of more elemental phenomena. Prestige is given to an explanation of behavior of a living organism in terms of responses to external stimuli, biochemical tensions, DNA composition and structure, etc.–in other words, *downward-looking* explanation.

Yet it is clear that scientists also use (often reluctantly) *upward-looking* explanation–explanation in terms of concepts at a higher level. For example, when the immune system attacks a particular virus it is not understood as just a complex chemical reaction; it can only be really understood in terms of the *function* of the immune system being to protect the organism from harm (a level-2 concept). In regeneration of a lobster claw after amputation, the complex building process can only be understood in terms of some kind of morphogenetic image of the nature of a whole lobster claw. To understand altruistic behavior it is necessary to invoke at least level-3, and possibly level-4, concepts. Teleological explanation (in terms of purpose or goal) is only one form of upward-looking explanation.

At the same time we recognize the validity of both downward-looking and upward-looking explanations, we need to note that the basic hunger for meaning, for making sense out of our lives, which is so characteristic of the human condition, tends to be more satisfied by the upward-looking explanations. They may or may not be more fundamental by some rational argument, but they *feel* more fundamental.

METHODOLOGY. The methodology used is that appropriate to a given level, and may be quite different for a different explanatory level. The rigidly controlled experiment, and the expectation of strict reliability of experimental results, are appropriate to the physical level and, to a more limited extent, the organismic. Even at these levels there may be intrusions of observer effect which are understandable from higher levels but "anomalous" at the lower.

The idea that the scientific observer cannot be "objective" in the sense of isolating himself completely from the phenomena observed applies at all levels to some extent, and particularly at the higher ones. What the scientist perceives is a function of unconscious conditioning and previous suggestions picked up from the environment. Furthermore, as the universe is perceived from the higher levels, the contents and processes of the experimenter's mind can affect the experiment in ways not understandable from the lower explanatory levels.

These kinds of considerations become especially relevant whenever "consciousness as causal reality" is a significant factor in the phenomena being observed. They suggest that strict interpretations of objectivity and of reliability through replicability are inappropriate in research on subjective experience. But surely, if they are, there must be other criteria something like these which <u>are</u> appropriate. Perhaps as the scientific exploration of these areas becomes more mature, something like the Buddhist idea of "nonattachment" will replace the concept of strict objectivity which, as is well known, no longer seems to fit even the relatively dependable area of the physical sciences. And something like "trustworthiness" (perhaps established on the basis of multiple imperfect tests) may replace strict reliability through replicability.

Consider as an example some of the recent work on multiple personalities. Is it really true that, incredible as it may seem at first thought, the same body may be inhabited by more than one personality? This holistic concept can hardly be explored at all without interacting with the person(s); thus objectivity in any strict sense is inappropriate. However, the ideal of nonattachment to preconceived notions of what can and cannot be is clearly pertinent. Not too long ago, the concept of an alternative personality expressing itself through the same body depended almost entirely on the psychiatrist's impressions. The concept has gained credibility in recent years because of the discovery that when the personality shifts, various measures of bodily functioning (e.g. fundamental voice characteristics; chemical composition of body fluids; allergic reactions) also change.

One other methodological point is important to note. In carrying out research that involves higher explanatory levels, the observer is not unchanged by his scientific

activities. One cannot explore altered states of consciousness without being sensitized and otherwise changed in the
process.

It is also the case that a willingness to be transformed
is an essential characteristic of the scientist of the higher
explanatory levels. The cultural anthropologist who would
see clearly another culture than his own must allow that
experience to change him so that the new culture is seen
through new eyes, not eyes conditioned by the scientist's
own culture. The psychotherapist who would see clearly
her client must have worked through her own neuroses
which would otherwise warp perception. The scientist who
would study at the level we have called "spiritual science"
has to be willing to go through the changes that will make
him/her a competent observer.

A CONCLUDING COMMENT

The importance of the issues raised here can hardly be
overestimated. It can be indicated by one simple sentence.
We in modern society give tremendous prestige and power
to our official, publicly validated knowledge system, namely
science. It is unique in this position; none of the other
coexisting knowledge systems—not any system of philosophy
or theology, nor philosophy or theology as a whole—is in a
comparable position. Thus the criticality of our science
being adequate is unparalleled. *It is impossible to create a
well-working society on a knowledge base which is fundamentally inadequate, seriously incomplete, and mistaken
in basic assumptions.* Yet that is precisely what the
modern world has been trying to do.

If one takes seriously the implication that Western
science is an artifact of Western society, based on implicit
assumptions compatible with that society's basic reality
outlook, it follows that the primary impetus for a fundamental change in its underlying assumptions will come not
from scientists, but from the surrounding culture. Indeed,

we see much evidence over the past quarter century that such a force may be gathering. Thus in writing this critique we are speaking as much to the public at large as we are to the scientist.

With this in mind, we have deliberately kept this argument simple, and minimized the amount of supportive detail and qualifications. The basic concept is a simple one, and can be understood by non-scientists. The cost of past dogma-versus-dogma conflicts, within and outside science, has been too high. It can no longer be afforded. The remedy may be to promote something like the hierarchically arranged explanatory levels suggested herein. It would certainly seem preferable to continued conflict over the evolution issue, the parapsychology issue, the vitalism issue, the holism/reductionism issue, the science-versus-religion issue, and so on ad infinitum.

(I would like to thank the many people whose writings and conversations have contributed to my thinking on this subject, including particularly my colleagues Morris Berman, Thomas Hurley III, Barbara McNeill, Brendan O'Regan, and Reneé Weber.)

REFERENCES

Berman, Morris, *The Reenchantment of the World*. Cornell University Press, 1981.

Koestler, Arthur, *Beyond Reductionism*. Beacon Press, 1971.

Kuhn, Thomas, *The Structure of Scientific Revolutions*, 2nd edition. University of Chicago Press, 1970.

Needleman, Jacob, *A Sense of the Cosmos*. E. P. Dutton, 1976.

Polanyi, Michael, *Personal Knowledge*. University of Chicago Press, 1958.

Sperry, Roger, "Changing Priorities". *Annual Review of Neurosciences*, (1981), pp. 1-10.

WELCOME

Remarks - Welcome

by

Kristie Knutson and Dr. Onslow H. Wilson

KRISTIE KNUTSON: My name is Kristie Knutson and I am the Master of Ceremonies for today's event. I am the Public Relations Director for the Rosicrucian Order. And as Master of Ceremonies it is my pleasure to be the very first to welcome you to the Annual Metaphysiology Symposium. This year the theme focuses on the "Mind As Healer."

It is particularly appropriate that the sponsor of this symposium is the Rosicrucian Order, AMORC. Over literally centuries, at times when it was not popular, this organization has been passionately devoted to exploring and developing the understanding and the full expression of human potential. As we discover and re-discover over and over again throughout the centuries, it is through the path of understanding the relationship between mind and body that we discover the true, full expression of this potential.

We have a very impressive panel of speakers with us today and I will be introducing each one of them to you individually before they speak. However, before we begin, I do want to share with you the fact that we have one program change. Unfortunately, it was not possible for Brendan O'Regan to be with us today [in San Jose.

However, he did address the Pasadena Symposium. See Chapter Five]. Nevertheless we are fortunate to have with us in his stead, Dr. Martin Rossman, who is with the Collaborative Medical Center and was specifically recommended by Mr. O'Regan himself.

To begin today's program, I am very pleased to introduce to you our first speaker, Dr. Onslow Wilson. Dr. Wilson is currently the Director of the Rosicrucian Order, AMORC's Department of Instruction. A biochemist, Dr. Wilson received his doctorate from McGill University in Montreal. He served as a post-doctoral fellow at the City of Hope Medical Center in Duarte, California. He later returned to Canada as Director of the Laboratory of Immunochemistry at the Clinical Research Institute of Montreal. He was also professor of Chemistry at Montreal's Dawson College. Dr. Wilson is the author of *Glands - The Mirror of Self*. Please join me in welcoming Dr. Onslow Wilson.

ONSLOW WILSON: Good morning. As you can see it has been a little harrowing this morning. But I, too, wish to extend my welcome to you on behalf of the Chief Executive Officer of this organization, Mr. Ralph M. Lewis who, unfortunately, cannot be with us today. As Kristie indicated, we are very proud to be sponsoring a symposium such as this because for years we have been interested in, and working feverishly at, this type of thing. We are, quite naturally, very pleased to see that the scientific community is now beginning to pay some attention to these areas. But we are not here to brag. Instead, I would like to give you a little background about this symposium—how it came to be.

About nine months ago, I was fortunate enough to have Dr. Willis Harman join me on a television program that AMORC sponsors, called "Ockham's Razor." My boss doesn't like the title, but I think it's an appropriate title because in the program we try to cut through the rye. At any rate, Dr. Harman indicated that it would be nice if we could participate in some sort of collaborative venture. Lo and behold, a few days later the seeds spawned in my mind that maybe we could have a symposium. But what were we going to call it? And so, after some thought we coined the phrase Metaphysiology. Again my boss cringed! But I would like to think that in years to come, when you turn to the dictionary to look up the term Metaphysiology, you will find the following definition: "The study of that aspect of mind which, directly or indirectly, impacts the physiology and biochemistry of the body." And that is precisely what we are here to look at today.

We have planned for you a very packed program, and so we are going to try to stick to schedule. We have organized everything as far as we can control. However, we are still in the process of negotiating with the "people upstairs" about the weather [it was threatening to rain]. These negotiations are important because we have planned a lunch—it's a catered affair—which we hope to have outside. We also have a string quartet which we also hope to enjoy outside. So the negotiations continue. And, hopefully, we will have a wonderful day during which we can enjoy the weather outside and the beautiful grounds that Rosicrucian Park has here. And with that, I welcome you once more. I turn you over now to Kristie Knutson. You will have much more to hear from me later, because I am the moderator for today's general discussions. And please, we want you to understand that the general discussions are basically organized for your benefit. We want you to feel free to participate; we want you to ask your questions, and we hope that we will be able to answer them for you. So please do participate. Once again, welcome. And now back to Kristie.

Chapter One

A NEW HERESY - A NEW MINDSET

by

Willis Harman, Ph.D.

KRISTIE KNUTSON: To begin the substance of today's program, I am very pleased to introduce to you our next speaker. Dr. Willis Harman is indeed in the tradition of the finest spirit of the renaissance scientist. He is President of the Institute of Noetic Sciences which, of course, was founded in 1973 by Edgar Mitchell, the astronaut. Dr. Harman is also Senior Social Scientist at Stanford Research Institute International; is Professor of Engineering Economics Systems at Stanford University; and is a member of the Board of Regents of the University of California. Throughout the 1960s, Dr. Harman was very active in the newly formed Association of Humanistic Psychology. Through his writings, among them, *An Incomplete Guide to the Future*, Dr. Harman has made a very profound impact on many of us. Please join with me now in welcoming Dr. Willis Harman.

WILLIS HARMAN: Thank you very much. It's my privilege to lead off this very interesting day. As you have inferred from the program, we know and recognize that it was not too many years ago that we wouldn't have had a symposium like this. In fact, it was not too long before that, that we probably wouldn't have talked about this subject very much because it has not always been popular.

Back in the middle of the nineteenth century, there were some operations performed in London and also in Calcutta, amputations and various kinds of major operations, using hypnotic suggestion as anesthesia. And these were done semi-publicly, that is, any member of the medical profession could observe. Medical journals in India, England and the United States all declined to publish the results on the grounds that there was no mechanism by which you could imagine the mind eliminating the pain and, therefore, this must be fraud and collusion; people must just have been pretending they didn't feel any pain while their legs were cut off and their bellies were slit open.

We look back on that, and it is rather amusing, but all the way along there have been topics, areas of human experience, that didn't fit into the currently popular way of looking at things. And it was sort of taboo to talk about those or to take them very seriously. A lot of these things we now accept as at least phenomena, even though we don't know what to do with them.

For example, hypnotic suggestion can raise various kinds of blisters that are pretty good imitations of blisters that come with different kinds of illnesses or with burns. This is a recognized phenomenon, even though we don't have much of an explanation yet, of course, for any of the aspects of hypnosis, especially for the basic phenomenon that the way you see the world is the way you have been hypnotized to see it. That's true when the suggestions came from a person called a hypnotist. It's equally true if the suggestions came from your culture, which is sort of the master hypnotist of all of us.

In that culture, in that particular way of looking at the world when we were going through a particular period in the history of science, it was not fashionable to think about the power of the mind creating illness, psychosomatic illness. We now recognize it and we now have a name for it, so that makes a lot of difference. We can now call it stress, and stress is something that creates psychosomatic illness and now it's all right to talk about it. It's still a bit mysterious, and so is the placebo effect where the influence of the mind is such that a chemical which really has no physiological effect, nevertheless, ends up healing an illness because we believe that it will.

A more controversial area is the use of imagery in affecting the functioning of the body's immune system. We'll be talking about a number of these things in more detail later on, but children can do this particularly well. In fact, children are so good at raising the body temperature, for example, that you can ask a little child to imagine that his finger is in a candle flame; to imagine the skin getting hotter and hotter—it's burning, it's feeling hotter and hotter—and the skin temperature goes up to 105 or 106 degrees, whereas the blood temperature remains at 98.6. Now adults can't seem to do that very well because they know it's impossible. But with children you can give the suggestion that they can imagine the body's immune system, and that they can imagine these little cells going around inside the body, sort of like Pac-Man, and chomping on the invaders in the body. The image doesn't have to be accurate, it just has to be one you can believe in. You can take a blood sample before this imaging exercise and observe the mobility of the white blood cells, then you can take another blood sample afterward (providing you have satisfied the Human Subjects Committee that this is really all right) and you can find that the immune cells do indeed seem to be noticeably more effective because of this imaging exercise. Now that is less controversial than the healing of cancer and other kinds of illness by imagining the body's immune system to be more effective.

Remission is a very puzzling sort of phenomenon because it is well known that people who have cancer and other life-threatening illnesses sometimes change their minds, sometimes decide not to die after all and the various symptoms disappear. We have a rather major project on this in the Institute of Noetic Sciences [see Chapter Five]. We started out by simply looking at the literature to see how much of this really is going on and it's far more than is ever talked about, and we are quite convinced that if we start talking about it, it will be more still. So there is an assortment, a rather wide assortment, of phenomena relating to the relationship between mind and healing that we're only now beginning to talk about openly and we recognize they don't really fit into the belief system of the past, the scientific belief system of the past. We are gradually getting comfortable with them and, of course, that scientific belief system is capable of some expansion. Now these phenomena of course don't all have to do with healing, they have to do with ordinary everyday sorts of things.

The two great mysteries about the human mind, if you look at it in certain ways, are the two phenomena of volition and attention. You know what it is to decide to do something; you know what it is to decide to pay attention. And yet in a certain sense, there is not only no scientific explanation for these, but there isn't any hope of one because the conscious decision-making mind has been ruled out of the picture from the start. Now that is a peculiar state of affairs where things that we know are part of human experience are defined as not part of science, but at the same time, we claim that science is our uniquely successful way of looking at the world. That's not a situation that's likely to last and it's not lasting. The basic phenomenon of human conscious awareness is not something that we are accustomed to talking about scientifically. I recently had lunch with the Chancellor of U.C. San Diego, who also is the author of one of the most successful psychology textbooks. And he told me with some pride that it is now going into its seventeenth edition and for the first time they have a chapter on consciousness.

When I studied science, I was encouraged to try to believe that conscious awareness was some kind of illusion. I was so impressed with my professors that I tried very hard to believe that. And I tried very hard to believe also that all these miraculous capabilities of the body's immune system and the other functioning parts of the body, all of those, evolved out of a long evolutionary process, physical, material evolution, by a process of random mutations and natural selection. So we end up having two eyes and binocular vision because some animal, by one of these chance occurrences, turned up with two eyes and had more survival capabilities than the animals with only one eye. I believed it! I can't believe myself, looking back, that I could swallow something like that. But you know, you'll do almost anything to get those degrees.

Creativity: we are all aware that there is some sort of mysterious, behind-the-scenes process. You can turn a problem over to it and wait an appropriate length of time and sure enough it comes up with some sort of a response, often a very good one. And again, the major advances in scientific conceptualization have been through this kind of creative, intuitive process; however, it's only very recently that there has been any attempt to deal with it in a scientific way.

Another interesting area that has just come to the fore in rather recent years is the study of multiple personalities. Now multiple personalities, of course, have been thought about pathologically for a long time. And most of us would consider it would be quite a misfortune to have had such abuse in early childhood that our personalities were fragmented, and at various times in the day different personalities come in and take over the same body.

The reason this became of interest again was because it turned out that when the personality shifts, not only are there changes in physiognomy and posture, and voice characteristics and so on, which had been known for a long time, but it also turns out that there are changes in the physiology of the body, changes in the chemical composition of the body fluids. The body may have certain allergies when one personality is in. When another personality takes over, the allergies disappear. In one case the body had a severe astigmatism with one personality, and when another personality came in the person could see perfectly.

Diabetic tendencies [are] the same way. So this becomes very interesting that a personality is a holistic kind of characteristic that you have to deal with, even though you can't measure it in the same sense that you can measure certain other kinds of scientifically treated variables. Well, all of this kind of ferment, inside and outside the scientific community, has led to a kind of reassessment about what are some of the fundamental assumptions underlying any consideration of the mind and healing, and all of these other interesting and somewhat mysterious aspects of life.

And so, I would like to spend the few minutes that we have together here, reminding or informing you of some of the things out on the front edge of that and make a guess as to where this is all going. Now even the concept of the unconscious mind is really one which has only recently been accepted in the scientific world.

I mean the world of hard science—you know, the kind that you can find at Stanford and Berkeley and the major research universities. The concept of the unconscious mind was questioned very seriously in that community. What apparently put it across were some studies on the phenomenon of subliminal perception. You are all familiar with these stories about subliminal perception.

The myth, of course, is that if you flash some pictures of popcorn and Coke on the screen in the movie house very briefly so you don't realize that you have even seen anything, nonetheless, you will get hungry and thirsty and go out in the lobby and start spending your money. But when this phenomenon was looked into more seriously, it turns out that there are some measurable characteristics in the brain that indicate that even when you're not consciously aware of having had this excitation by the short flash of a picture, nonetheless, if the picture is one that would produce some sort of emotional response, it tends to produce something like that anyway.

Not only that, but the indications from your response to this picture are that unconsciously you must have seen the picture, recognized the pattern, recognized whatever words may have been there, performed some kind of semantic analysis, understood the meaning to you, and responded—all without any participation by the conscious mind! Well, for many of us I suppose the reality of the unconscious mind is just something that is part of our experience. It betrays itself in all sorts of ways, but it is now a recognized scientific concept.

There is another experiment that I would like to briefly describe to you because it also has a powerful implication with regard to what's going on that must now be taken into account in any sort of scientific story about how reality operates. This is Ernest Hilgard's rather well-known by now Ice Pail Experiment, in which a person is hypnotized to not feel pain in, say, the left hand—to feel no pain in the left hand when it is put into a bucket of ice cubes.

Now if you ever have put your hand into a bucket of ice water you would realize that there is excruciating pain after just a short time. So the person holds the hand in [the ice cubes] and insists he or she feels no pain because that's what the mind believes.

Meanwhile, with the gaze averted to somewhere, in some other direction, the person is invited to take a pen in the right hand and just let the hand go—do automatic writing just let it scrawl out whatever it wants to on a piece of paper. So here is the person with the left hand sitting in this bucket of ice water and the right hand writing things like, "Ouch! It hurts! Stop it!" So apparently we're all multiple personalities. Professor Hilgard called this particular entity behind the scenes the hidden observer.

Now we are culturally hypnotized to see the world in a way that is different from the way that other cultures see it. So in some cultures there is the phenomenon of fire-walking that's taken for granted. Certain people in a certain state of mind can walk barefoot over burning coals and not hurt their feet. Now the last two or three years, literally thousands of well-educated people in this country, in professional and business positions, have gone through this fire-walking episode. In fact, we required it of our board members a year ago. I mean that literally—we did. You stand in front of this fire and you can tell from the way the heat hits your face, that if you put a steak on there, it's not going to hesitate with regard to starting the barbecuing process.

But, nevertheless, if you hold your mind a certain way, you step out on those coals, and it's cool and comfortable and it doesn't do anything serious to the flesh. On the other hand, you hold your mind another way, whatever that means, and it's not even easy to describe, and you barbecue your feet. So here is a phenomenon which, until the last few years, did not seem to be even possible—not conceivable—in our culture, and yet it was an everyday occurrence in certain other cultures.

Now I'm quite familiar with all the arguments about the thin layer of ash that insulates your feet and all that stuff, and if you want to go into that, we can, but there is a real phenomenon here in spite of all explaining away that has been done, and it's as mysterious as all these other things that we've been talking about.

Another example is the remote viewing used for military intelligence in the U.S. and U.S.S.R.—the phenomenon of sending your mind out some distance to see what's going on, hundreds or thousands of miles, to see which silo the MX missile is in and all that sort of thing. But it was not very long ago in our culture that we did not believe anything like that was possible. And as a matter of fact the only research funding that has gone into it in any major way has indeed been from the military.

I think it might be worth describing one of these experiments. This is one that was done in Stanford Research Institute among other places, just to give you the feel for what a mysterious thing this is. In this experiment, the person who has practiced and seems to be capable of accomplishing this phenomenon, is given two randomly chosen numbers. Now one of those numbers is the latitude and the other one is the longitude. So together they represent the intersection of two lines somewhere on the surface of the earth.

Nobody knows where that spot is because the numbers were randomly chosen. The person is asked to send your mind out to that spot, see what's there, come back and make a sketch, and then we'll compare it using complicated judging procedures. We'll compare it with the photograph in that spot. Now it turns out the person is able to do this. And it's very hard to think of a so-called mechanism by which that could be accomplished.

The most interesting thing about all of this work on remote viewing is that when you train someone to do this, the main element in the training is getting rid of the negative belief that you can't do it, because unconsciously you already know how. Just as unconsciously, you already know how to raise the skin temperature to 106 degrees, and you know how to create stomach ulcers, and you know how to heal stomach ulcers, and all the rest.

Unconsciously, we believe just as we believe consciously; unconsciously we make choices; unconsciously we perform analyses; unconsciously we think we know things we don't know we know consciously. What goes on in the conscious mind is only the tiniest tip of the iceberg. Now it happens to be about ninety-nine percent of what we're concerned with in that activity we call education. That may change sometime too.

But here we know this is true. There is no question about the vast majority of our mental activity going on outside conscious awareness. There is no question any more about the fact that our lives are far more affected, our perceptions, our behaviors, our values, are far more affected by what's going on in the unconscious part of the mind, than they are by the conscious part.

And yet, we don't take that seriously by-and-large. That, again, is something that we're just beginning to take more seriously. As a matter of fact, if you look carefully at some of the courses that are being given for management development, executive training, and so on, you'll find that, although in our formal education we don't pay any attention to this in the schools and universities, in executive development they pay a great deal of attention to it these days in spite of the fact that the phenomena that you're involved with there, again, don't fit in.

For example, executives are trained to realize that they can change their unconscious programming; they can change the unconscious beliefs by a process of affirmation or inner imagery. Now this is something that has been known in Christian Science circles and elsewhere for a long, long time, but it's fairly new to the business world and it's even newer to the scientific world if you push it very far.

It's not clear that there are any limits to the power of the mind to imagine a result already being accomplished and then sit back and watch the universe set out to accomplish it. Now that sounds like spooky kind of talk

for executives. You know, after all, they are the essence
of practicality. Nevertheless, that is what they are talking
about these days. And of course in all of the world's
spiritual traditions, this has been known for a long time
and in the Christian formulation one of the most familiar
expressions of it is, "Whatever you pray for, believe that
you'll receive it, and you will." Whatever it is you want
to image, hold that image, and in mysterious ways it will
tend to come about. Well, how are we going to handle
that scientifically?

Another lesson that executives are trained in is that
there is no necessity for fear. There is no necessity for
fear of failure, fear of criticism, fear of ridicule, fear of
success, all the things that typically get in our way. The
only reason you fear anything is because you believe it is
fearful. Change the unconscious beliefs by an affirmation
process, change the perceptions in that sense, and you
don't perceive anything fearful and you don't fear anymore—a very practical lesson! But it doesn't fit in.

The first person of Nobel laureate stature who announced
publicly and bravely and maybe in a foolhardy way that we
have to do something about these areas that don't fit
in—the first person, I think, was Roger Sperry in about
1982, in an article entitled "Changing Priorities." He said
in essence, "We've had the most amazing blind spot in
science and we didn't recognize it." We didn't realize
there was a whole neglected area that we weren't dealing
with—the area of human inner subjective experience.
Whatever was done with that was really relatively trivial
compared to the vastness of the territory and compared to
the thoroughness with which science explores other areas
of a more material sort.

Sperry is the one, you recall, who gave us the right and
left brain conceptualization that has done so much for pop
psychology. He said, "This is a tremendously important
area that we have neglected because all lives and all
societies guide themselves by some kinds of value commit-

ments, some kinds of sense of meaning, that we all get from our deep inner experience."

So if we neglect this area as a culture, it can have disastrous consequences and it probably is. So we find then, in his suggestion—and he's not the only one by now, another Nobel laureate, Sir John Eccles in England, and various others, have been saying the same thing—that we have to deal not only with the world that physicists deal with (which is the world of matter-energy, that is, the fundamental stuff in the universe is matter-energy; they are convertible, and we can explore this down to the properties of the most elementary particles, and when we do, we run into some amazing things, such as particles which are very distant from one another, seemingly nevertheless, in contact with one another), you have to deal with the universe as a whole.

But nevertheless, we don't learn a whole lot beyond that because physics is essentially a reductionistic science still, but at least it has demonstrated the limits of reductionistic science. So we have to go somehow beyond the world of matter-energy. We have to get beyond the point of insisting that the only thing that's real is the physical and chemical processes in the brain and that consciousness, mind, and spirit don't have any reality in a scientific sense.

Now very few scientists have spoken out as boldly as this. They either have to be very young and not really care, or they have to be old enough to have tenure, but you see what's happening. If you go back to the seventeenth century, there was a heresy abroad. It turns out to have been a very important heresy: it changed the world.

Heresy is when you say, "You know the world is not the way the authorities have been telling us." And in this case, it was the church authority. Now that particular heresy we call the scientific revolution. It was so profound that the world that was seen by an educated person in the year 1700, was totally different from the world literally seen by the person in 1600.

Now we associate certain key figures for this: Copernicus, Galileo, and so on, but in fact it looks as though there was a lot of discontent with what the authorities had been claiming. But that discontent didn't surface very much until there was something it could hang on to. So when Copernicus came forth with this idea of the earth traveling around the sun, there was a sudden surge of getting on board. And so a change in mindset all over Western Europe took place very rapidly. And it really amounted to a shift in the kind of authority that you assume is the last word. It was a shift from the traditional authority, particularly the authority of the church; it was a shift from that over to the authority of what we now call empirical science.

Now for political and psychological reasons, as science started out, it adopted a couple of metaphysical assumptions that turned out to be very important. I'm giving you, obviously, a rather simplified history, but that's all we have time for in a few minutes, and it's not too distorted.

The fundamental assumptions of science were, first of all, what is scientifically real is what is physically measurable—the so-called positive assumption. And the other one was the assumption that the kinds of explanations you were seeking are explanations in terms of complicated phenomena explained in terms of simple ones—the reductionistic assumption. So if I want to explain human behavior, I think of it in terms of the glandular secretions and the mechanical forces and things of that sort or maybe ultimately in terms of how the electrons and the atoms are moving around in the fields.

That's what we mean by an explanation. There is no concept of purpose, there's no concept of explanations in terms of people or evolutionary processes trying to go somewhere, trying to go in a particular direction. That was ruled out. Now this was partly because of division of territory. That is, the fledgling scientific group had an implicit agreement with the church that the church could take care of the inner life and the scientist would deal with the outer world.

Nonetheless, those assumptions really resulted in a tremendous success story because they are exactly the assumptions you need if what you want to do is generate a knowledge system that can create fascinating new technologies for putting a man on the moon, and creating new organisms, and all the other fascinating things we can do these days. It was just exactly right for that, but science as it developed is a lousy guide to life and to guiding societies because it essentially says there aren't any meanings and purposes by which to guide yourself.

Now that's a temporary thing. As a matter of fact, we've already passed through the peak of that. It was about a half century ago that we really believed and taught in our schools positivism and reductionism. There is this new heresy abroad and it's potentially just as important and just as fundamental in its society-changing capabilities as was the scientific revolution. This new heresy doesn't have a name yet. But in essence, [just] as the scientific revolution amounted to saying that the world was not the way the church authorities had been telling us, the new heresy is saying that the world is not the way the secular authorities have been telling us either. And so it's only really in the last few years that you've heard people of high educational attainment, and in high positions in the society, saying anything like that. And I don't think they've heard about it yet in the academic world.

Now, in the world's spiritual traditions there is a tradition of research. Research has been going on for a long, long time in laboratories that are called monasteries. And some of the thought-systems that have come out of this are amazingly sophisticated. But the most important thing that has developed out of studies of the different spiritual traditions in the world (and remember, comparative religion is essentially a new discipline within the last half century; prior to that nobody really cared because we already knew which one was best) . . . [is that] you find that they tend to have public versions and then esoteric, inner-circle versions.

The public versions differ a great deal one from the other. They have different rituals and differently shaped temples, and different kinds of beliefs and so on. The inner-circle, esoteric versions are much more based on human experience. They tend to be associated with some kind of discipline, a meditative discipline, yoga or something like that. And they tend to be more or less the same. They tend to be saying that if you look deeply within, you'll come more or less to the same place that you would come to if you had been in some other tradition and you follow similar kinds of spiritual disciplines.

In that perennial wisdom, the world is full of consciousness; the world is full of purpose. If we ask why do we behave the way that we do, we don't think in terms of an explanation, in terms of our genetic inheritance plus whatever we have learned, whatever behavior-shaping has happened along the way, we have to think of genes plus behavior plus something else, and that something else has to do with consciousness, mind, spirit. Learning is not learning knowledge from the outside alone. In fact, it's not even that mainly. The really important kind of learning is remembering what you already know—in this belief system.

Now this belief system is very, very different from the one that has dominated the Western world and has tended then to dominate the whole globe. And I want to just give two examples of how different it really is. One is the story of evolution and the other is the story of what's real. Now in the story of evolution, in the conventional picture that we have of this, the neo-Darwinist picture, there seems to have been about fifteen billion years ago a

Big Bang, and everything started—at least everything in this universe that we know.

Then there was the evolution of stars and planets, and elementary life forms and animals and, finally, the human being. Various processes of random mutation and natural selection were going on, and then we finally get to this point where the neuronal cells in the brain are so numerous and the inner connections are so complex, that we have this phenomenon of human consciousness. Then we try to explain that in terms of various kinds of computer operations in the brain or something like that, but at any rate, we do recognize we have consciousness, we do pay attention, we do choose to act and so on. Now that's more or less the story: the conventional scientific one. Now alongside that, there's the creationist story. And as you know the Supreme Court is to decide which of these stories is right for America sometime this fall because of a Louisiana law that is insisting that if you are going to teach neo-Darwinism you have to teach Creationism alongside of it, and we're going to decide whether that's constitutional or not.

In fact, it really doesn't make too much difference which story the Supreme Court is in favor of, since they're both wrong anyway, or at least since they're both incomplete. And what seems to be the more accurate story, or the one that seems to fit all that we know—all the scientific knowledge and also the knowledge of this perennial wisdom of the world's spiritual traditions—the story seems more to be one like fifteen billion years ago there was a Big Bang and all the rest of this and, finally, we have human consciousness, **but, consciousness was there in the universe all along**, and it was pulling the evolutionary process at the same time that it was being pushed by natural selection.

Now that isn't such a big shift but, nonetheless, in its implications it probably is a very big shift. Just as when fundamental assumptions changed during the scientific revolution, they really changed everything, all the institutions of the society, this one is at the same level. If the assumptions change at this level, what it really means is since everything is now speeded up quite a bit, the world of the twenty-first century is going to be as different from the modern world as the modern world is from the middle ages. So it makes a lot of difference whether what I am telling you really stands up or doesn't.

Let me just give the other example that will illustrate again how different is the conventional scientific worldview from this expanded scientific worldview, which is of a more metaphysical sort, but which does not contradict the scientific world at all. It simply says, "Well it is incomplete, let us expand the boundaries and then do something else with it." In trying to compare these two, let us think of this metaphysical perennial wisdom view in the following analogy.

You have a dream, and in that dream, there's a story line of some sort, various events happen, and they seem to cause other events and so on. It all seems very real, and then you wake up. You look back and say, well the law of causality is not what I thought it was when I was dreaming. It's now clear that I, the dreamer, caused all the events and all the relationships and hence the real causality is that I, the dreamer, caused the whole dream.

Now, here we are in this reality situation, the chairs feel real and you all seem real to one another, and there seem to be various causal relationships in all of this. And some of those causal relationships seem to happen so regularly that we call them scientific laws. You know if I drop an object it usually falls to the floor. That's a scientific law. Once in a while there may be an exception, but then we don't pay much attention to that. So here's this world, but every so often somebody wakes up, they call it "enlightenment." Every so often somebody wakes up and looks back and says, you know the law of causality is not what we thought it was. I, we, the collective dreamer, with our minds all interconnected, we create this dream we call reality, this world of matter-energy. And so it's not so surprising that once in a while you seem to see exceptions to the positivistic, reductionistic picture, since that's just a partial picture anyway.

What I've been really trying to say in this limited time that we have together, is that I believe there are lots and lots of signs that we are at a very fateful point in history. And I mean it literally when I pick out the scientific revolution as the last great heresy that we remember, and suggest that by comparison we have another heresy right now, and it probably is going to make as much difference as that [last revolution].

In this, what seems to be emerging is a belief-system, and this seems to be emerging very rapidly. I picked out the executive development courses to call those to your attention, because we have so much respect for the pragmatic practicality of the world of business; they do not wait until we have all the niceties of the scientific theories worked out; they just say, you know if it works let's use it; we'll figure it out later. It does seem to work.

I can show you executive development seminars where they literally teach: Do not believe there are any limits. Do not believe there are any limits to the ability of affirming and changing the unconscious programming in your mind; do not believe there are any limits to the effects that can be had in the outer external world. Because if you believe there are limits, they will be there, and so, since you don't know what the limitations are, don't believe in any.

Similarly, we don't know what the limitations are of the mind as regards to healing the body and healing the psyche, therefore it is safer not to believe in any limitations. And not very long ago that would have been considered to be an unscientific statement, or even an anti-scientific statement! Now we are on the edge of the time in which it may be the most sophisticated kind of scientific statement that we can make. And so that kind of an orientation, if we believed it, could lead to a great deal of exhilaration about the rest of this day because now what we are about to explore are not some off-beat, hidden, dark corners that don't yet fit into the scientific worldview.

We are going to explore some phenomena and some experiences that are going to fit very quickly into an expanded kind of scientific worldview, which we have needed for some time and we've needed it not just to deal with healing the individual but with healing the planet. And things are happening very, very rapidly and shortly we will hear about it [a new worldview]. Thank you.

Chapter Two

THE NEW HERESY IN THE CORPORATE WORLD

by

Kenneth Pelletier, Ph.D.

KRISTIE KNUTSON: Thank you, Dr. Harman. It's my pleasure to introduce our second speaker today, Dr. Kenneth Pelletier. Dr. Kenneth Pelletier is an internationally recognized clinician, researcher and lecturer in holistic medicine and preventive health care. Dr. Pelletier is an Associate Clinical Professor of Internal Medicine and Psychiatry at the Langley-Porter Neuropsychiatric Institute in San Francisco. He's also an Associate Professor of Public Health at the University of California in Berkeley. He tells me that he can now feel free to speak out in the forefront of science because he did receive his tenure in July.

Dr. Pelletier has published over two hundred articles in professional journals in the areas of holistic medicine, psychosomatic medicine, stress, clinical biofeedback, and neurophysiology. His research and clinical practice have been the subject of many national TV programs including The Today Program, ABC World News and the award winning BBC Series, "The Long Search." Dr. Pelletier's works include *Mind as Healer/Mind as Slayer,* a holistic approach to preventing stress disorders. Please join me now in welcoming Dr. Pelletier.

KENNETH PELLETIER: Thank you and good morning. It's always nice to follow Willis Harman. In fact, as he was speaking, I remembered the first time I heard you [Dr. Harman] lecture nearly twenty years ago at a meeting of Congressional leaders at Early House in Virginia, and I was as moved then as I was this morning. You've always had a great influence on my thinking so whatever I'm about to say this morning is all your fault. [laughter]

I was very struck, as usual, with the visionary kind of presentation that you [Dr. Harman] mentioned, in particular, in work in the corporate sector with senior management. And that's precisely what I want to talk about this morning. [There are] really two studies, both of which are ongoing, and both of which I think demonstrate to me, day in and day out, how extraordinarily far we have come.

The two studies, one of which I'll show you in considerable detail on some slides, the two studies that are currently being conducted are both within the Department of Internal Medicine at the University of California School of Medicine in San Francisco. The one which . . . could perhaps be a very striking example of how far . . . the applications of mind/body technologies have come, is a current program where we are working with fifteen major corporations to develop and evaluate an array of what have been termed health promotion programs. These include stress management, behavioral management of hypertension, certain forms of cancer screenings, the use of meditative practices and visualization-like activities within the corporate environment for a very practical reason, which is [that they have] the effect of improving overall performance and productivity, and lowering medical claims and disabilities. It really is very bottom-line oriented.

Just to give you some idea, I think I would like to underscore the fact that this could hardly be considered esoteric. Let me just read you the names of the participating corporations: Apple Computer, AT&T, Bank of America, Bechtel (who has given us two prominent leaders recently) Chevron, Crown Zellerbach, Hewlett Packard, Levi, McKesson, PG&E, Pacific Telesis, Safeway, Shaklee, Southwestern Bell Corporation (which is the only one that's not in the Bay Area for some reasons that will be clear as we go along) and Wells Fargo Bank.

I think that's a fairly impressive array. We are in the second year of a five year program. It's rather a complicated program, but essentially what we're doing with these companies is creating a collaborative effort where we develop programs for them, apply them, and evaluate them both for health efficacy and for financial efficacy. So it's a serious effort to apply many of the technologies that we are considering this morning. And again, they really don't care about mediators. As a scientist, I find that somewhat difficult but nonetheless, I welcome [the opportunity] to be able to work in a context in which practicality and results are emphasized and they certainly are here.

The second study on which I want to give you some detail actually goes back to 1982. Now between 1982 and 1983 two things happened that we are all familiar with. One is that AT&T was divested or broken up. Practically speaking, it meant that we all now have bigger phone bills and less service. The second was that banking was deregulated. Now these are, predictably, times of extraordinarily high stress. In 1982, a group of us decided to do what was then a rather naive [piece of] research. . . . At this point we know on the basis of probably about twenty years of research that under conditions of stress, protracted stress, that if you take any large or small group of individuals, twenty percent of that group will manifest disease. So if we followed ourselves out over the next year, we would find that twenty percent of us would manifest virtually all of the disease for this group as a whole. That's . . . fairly predictable.

Also there is a subset of that group, roughly five to seven percent, that will actually die. Now we knew that, and given the enormous stress of divestiture and deregulation, you could predict that that would occur in banking and telecommunications. And it did! Now we asked a naive question and met with the medical directors and corporate personnel directors of the two most prominent representatives, AT&T and Bank of America. We said, what we would like to do is follow a select sample of your executives through this period of major transition to see if—and we didn't know if this were the case—to see if there was an equally small group, five to seven percent, who would not only not die or become ill, but [instead] would actually perform better, who would actually rise to the occasion, who would meet the challenge, who would represent states of optimal health and optimal performance.

In fact, it held out to be true. We did find that there were two groups of executives and this subgroup, this optimally healthy group, had very striking characteristics (approximately fifteen, some medical, some psychological and some managerial) which differentiated these two groups almost one hundred percent. And this morning we will look at a few of these.

The reason I can't go through the whole presentation is that, literally, it takes three hours . . . AT&T has always had a reputation of being a maternalistic, caring corporation which pays a lot of attention to the evolution of its corporate culture. You know it's called Ma Bell. And Ma Bell was just that: it was a very caring, maternalistically structured organization. They have a thing which they call their corporate policy seminars, their CPS. . . . By way of demonstrating how seriously they take the evolution of their corporate culture, they . . . actually take their roughly fifteen to sixteen hundred senior managers through an orientation seminar, fifty at a time.

It takes about thirty seminars in the course of a two-year interval to expose them to new ideas and evolve the viability of the corporation to meet the new world. These slides that you'll see bear the Bell logo because it was when it was still the integrated Bell System. [This is] the presentation that was used in the course of their management seminars and has subsequently been used in others of the now divested, or singular, corporations like Southwestern Bell Corporation of the AT&T Systems. It's about as practical as it could get.

So let me now back up just for one minute, and provide a context for seeing this because some of the specifics are important and they are going to be amplified in the course of the day. But I think to understand these large global trends, some of which Dr. Harman has referred to [is] . . . extremely important and not to be underestimated. Now just by way of a quick trajectory, most of my research from late 1960s to the mid-to late 1970s was concerned about the neurophysiological correlates by which mind and body could control, to extraordinary degrees, things we thought could not be controlled. And Joe Kamiya and myself, at the University of California—and in fact, our research was supported by the Institute of Noetic Sciences at the time, among some others—we studied a group of adept meditators during this interval, and some of you may be familiar with the work.

One of the participants was Jack Schwartz, a Dutch meditator who did interesting things like skewer his arm with large diameter knitting needles. When we looked at what was occurring on the electroencephalograph (the readings from the brain-wave activity) we found he was not experiencing pain. Other individuals we've studied, categorized as adept meditators, did not experience pain [either] even at the electrical level of activity. They did not bleed; they could voluntarily control bleeding. They could voluntarily control infection and they did not even have the basic kinds of reactions you might expect to deliberately induced infections that we would try to do with them. By the way, you could not even do this work anymore because of human subjects limitations, but we could then.

By 1974 there was beginning to develop a critical body of research which demonstrated that this mind/body interaction had extraordinary properties . . . which neither one alone could explain. Now one of the first quotes that struck me that this might be applicable in a practical kind of way was in 1974 [in] the New England Journal of Medicine, which is the most conservative of the AMA publications. If you want to know the absolute hard line, this is the journal you would choose to read, for those of us who are masochistic enough to read this thing. [laughter]

In 1974, the then chief editor, a Harvard trained surgeon (again, chief editor of the most conservative journal) was asked to write an editorial on the capacity of medical care to create health in the population as a whole. Create health! Now bear in mind this is at a time when we were spending 310 billion dollars [annually] on medical care in the United States.

This was the quote that was published in the 1974 New England Journal of Medicine. It says, "Let us assume that eighty percent of patients have either self-limited disorders or conditions not improvable even by modern medicine." Now that's not an impressionistic figure; it's the other side of the twenty percent that I stated earlier. "The doctor's actions, unless harmful, therefore do not affect the basic course of such conditions. In slightly over ten percent of cases, however, medical interventions have been dramatically successful." And it goes on to elaborate largely what we would call emergency room procedures, things that we do which are clearly diagnosed and have clear kinds of interventions.

The point being that this is not anti-scientific, it's not anti-medical, it's simply to recognize what is appropriate and what is not. "But alas in the final nine percent, give or take a point or two, the doctor may diagnose or treat inadequately or may just have bad luck." That's the line that I like. Whatever the reason, the patient ends up with atrogenic problems; the atrogenesis—that's if the disease doesn't get you the cure will.

In fact, we are beginning to realize that with seemingly benign interventions like anti-hypertensive medications or blood pressure medications the effects of these medications are not benign and are quite problematic. The National Institutes of Health has major grants, one of which we are working with, with Bank of America, to look at alternatives to pharmacological treatment because for many complex reasons, they are really problematic. Now the last line if you will: "So the balance of accounts ends up marginally on the positive side of zero." The most conservative estimate of the capacity of 310 billion dollars to buy health, is marginally on the positive side of zero! You can't do any worse.

What has evolved over the last twelve years is to some degree a measure which looks at what are the preconditions by which we produce optimal health, optimal performance and productivity. It is, in fact, in the domain of the automatization of mind/body interactions.

If we could come very rapidly up to the present time, let me read you two other things. In October of each year the Journal of the American Medical Association, probably the second most conservative publication, gives a retrospective on medical care for the prior year and looks toward the coming years. In the last one, which was in October of 1985, there were two statements both of which I'll read to you, which I think point to . . . [a] more optimistic, more positive direction which acknowledges in a practical way many of the same things we heard about earlier this morning.

This was a restatement of that position in 1974. Now I'd like to point out to you that now the annual medical expenditure is 450 billion dollars, and the statement I read in 1974 is still true. Perhaps even more so, as you'll see with this next one. This was the statement: "About two-thirds"—keep track of these figures—"About two-thirds of all deaths in this country are premature given our present medical knowledge." Not some biotechnological break-through [but] present medical knowledge. . . . "About two-thirds of all years of life lost before age sixty-five are preventable given our current capabilities." Now that's astounding! This is part of the reason why, at least for me, the most intriguing question has not become if, or how, or what are the mediators, but how do we apply what in fact we have known for decades, if not fifty or sixty years or perhaps longer.

So the intriguing question is, What can we do about this extraordinary misuse or misdirection (in a very practical way) that impacts us day in and day out?

Now given the enormous complexity of this problem, what begins to look like a solution? The ironic thing is that the solution is not as complex as the problem, for-tunately. And in fact, later in that same issue of the Journal of the American Medical Association comes the basis, or at least the trajectory, for a possible beginning of a solution.

Let me interject in here [that] shortly after that October statement in the Journal of the American Medical Associa-tion which caused a great uproar, that did not get taken lightly, the New England Journal of Medicine (and perhaps some of you saw this because this was on virtually every national news broadcast) did a very heretical thing. This was I believe in February or March of 1986, so this is really quite current.

Two researchers, two epidemiologists at Harvard University Medical School, went to the National Cancer Institute and said, "You know we don't want to generate any new data to be accused of somehow biasing our analysis. You give us your data on morbidity and mortality from all forms of cancer, and we would like to then do some analyses on your data, [that of the] National Cancer Institute." What they found in analyzing the data . . . [from] between 1981 and 1985, (which had the largest and most unprecedented increase in cancer funding research and ostensible application) was that there was actually a five percent increase in overall cancer mortality. Now, the conclusion of this analysis, which was stated in the New England Journal [of Medicine] . . . said, "A shift in research emphasis from research on treatment to research on prevention seems necessary if substantial progress against cancer is to be forthcoming." That's astounding considering these sources.

Now, what would this look like? What would a possible solution look like? And I think this brings us directly to what the subject is today: "Mind as Healer," which sounds awfully familiar to me somehow [because of the book *Mind as Healer/Mind as Slayer* by Dr. Pelletier].

"The scientific basis for the influence of lifestyle choices on health continues to grow. Lifestyles are changing and these changes are already reducing the toll of diseases. We have had about a twenty percent decline in heart disease due virtually entirely to lifestyle choices and interventions. In the coming decades the most important determinants of health and longevity will be those personal choices made by each individual. This is both frightening for those who wish to avoid such responsibility and exciting for those who desire a measure of control over their own destinies." I think that's a wonderful statement [from *Mind as Healer/Mind as Slayer*].

Now as we look at these slides that we have developed, and are following these executives in banking and communications, bear in mind that these are individuals. . . . And I think it's a challenge to all of us who in practices, outlook, and impact on our world, have chosen to be active perpetrators. So what I would now like to briefly show you [are] a few of the initial slides which are presented in the course of these seminars.

Bear in mind . . . where these are being used. Now the initial slide I start off with is the oldest picture I could find of the physician [slide shown]. Actually it is a picture of the Greek root for physician, physis. And this is an illustration of the physis. If you could see this more clearly—let me describe it; just close your eyes and visualize this picture of the physis.

The physis has two definitions. One is an exoteric definition and it means nature. The initial function of the physis or the healer would be to harmonize the person with nature. It is symbolized by the color green, and the initial function would then be to bring a person into harmony with the universe.

This [other] is more accurately a description of the esoteric or the internal definition of the physis. . . . There is a person standing in the middle of this figure and the one thing that's most obvious is [that it is] a very hermaphroditic figure. It's a fusion of the male and female, the active, the passive, the left and right hemispheres of the brain, yin/yang. In other words, a picture of harmony, integration and balance is always an essential part of healing and optimal health. The person's right hand is holding a pitcher or a solution, a potion. At that time it probably would have been an herbal or perhaps a homeopathic remedy. The point is that medications or interventions, surgery, whatever, have a place. Technology, science, has an appropriate place in the healing traditions but it's not all that there is.

In the person's left hand is a book, a standard of practice, something that guides at least our current knowledge and gives us a point of departure for other and perhaps more encompassing approaches. Maybe it's the first century Merck Manual or something. Then the person is standing in the circle of the zodiac. There are some very embarrassing quotations which I like to use at medical meetings from Hippocrates, or the Hippocratic Oath, that, "The physician who does not know astrology should not be practicing." He meant that quite literally. For the Greek, the early Greek physicians, medicine and astrology were one and the same; no one would think of treating without doing the chart. Then there are the demonic elements, the two demon-like figures at the base, if you will, the psyche.

There is a fascinating new area of research called psychoneuroimmunology. It sounds rather complicated to say, but the "psycho" is the mind, "neuro" the brain and central nervous system, and "immunology" the body's own defense against viral or bacterial infection or the development of cancer, abnormal cells internally. This area has all the characteristics of a major breakthrough in understanding mind/body interactions that the structure of the DNA did in the 1950s. And I think that one particular project you [Dr. Harman] pointed to on spontaneous remission is just such an area.

Then there's the emphasis on the totality of the environment. So it is in fact a systemic, holistic approach that is at the root of the Western medical tradition . . . and in fact, in all healing traditions globally. So the point is, rather than seeing a systemic or a holistic approach as a deviation, in fact. . . pharmacological high-tech intervention is [the] deviation from tradition and we seem to be coming back the other way.

Now . . . to this [slide]. For those who cannot read the sign around the man's neck, it says $117.00 a day plus medication. This shows you what inflation has done. This slide's about five years old and when I found it, that was a lot of money. And at this point, that's the cost of your medication if you are in an HMO [Health Maintenance Organization].

This is simply a practical look at the impact of a high technology approach to chronic degenerative diseases which, in fact, can't be treated. So it's the wrong model, with manifest problems. Let me just show you that last one [slide] by way of one example. Xerox Corporation has one of the largest well-developed health promotion programs for both senior executives and main line employees. When I began working with them six years ago, the factor that got them moving was they were diversifying into a major new area of management and they had one young man age forty-one, who was in charge of that division, [and he] died of a sudden first event inexplicable coronary. At least on their terms . . . the estimated . . . direct cost, six or seven years ago, [was] one million dollars to replace that individual. So suddenly the cost of developing a series of health programs for management seemed quite trivial and has remained so.

Now what have we learned by tracking over 300 executives in banking? Some of the banks that are represented are Bank of America, Citicorp, Chase Manhattan; on the communication side [are] AT&T, Central Illinois Bell, Southwestern Bell Corporation and Pacific Telesis. What have we found? Now the interesting thing is [that] the first characteristics are really totally psychological, and turned out to be perhaps the most accurately predictive of a person's health and performance.

So these represent a point of psychological orientation, around which many of the practices and behaviors seem to constellate or spin off. It's not epiphenomenal to a set of behaviors; it is central, causative. It's the point of power; it's the point of personal empowerment which meditative practices have told us for literally centuries.

The first characteristic we found, called [one of] the three Cs, was challenge. Now the point of challenge is that these were the same set of external circumstances [for everyone]. These were divestiture and deregulation. Everyone was facing the same set of external circumstances. Now if a person perceived this external set of circumstances as overwhelming, as negative, as threatening, as outside of their control or influence, they began to succumb, get sick and die. By the way, that five to seven percent mortality was right on the head. Just that number of individuals died in the population that was being studied.

On the other hand, those individuals who chose volitionally to see the same set of external circumstances as a challenge to innovate [and who believed] something was going to change and this was an opportunity [said], "We can innovate, make a difference, etc." In other words, they found the excitement in these changing circumstances. [These] were the ones who survived, thrived, developed, etc.

The second [of the three Cs] was commitment. Now it's obviously different if you perceive a challenge versus whether you become committed or not. All of us might perceive a challenge in the rapidly changing paradigm and the rapidly changing world in which we're living. It's quite a different matter to get committed.

Now the opposite of commitment is to avoid and deny. "It's not real. This anomalous information both in basic science and application are somehow not real. We're going to wake up tomorrow and the world is going to be just the same as it has always been." So denial, removal, retreat, etc. are all the ways that these individuals began to deny the reality of having to adapt to the changing circumstances in their corporations and in their environment. The difference [was that] the ones who survived and thrived [had] a two-fold level of commitment. The most obvious one was on an external level where they got involved. They said, "I am going to take some chances. Here is an idea that I have. I am going to reconfigure my department, I am going to think up a new product, I am going to, in fact, be creative. I am going to think about what I can do advantageously in this new world."

Secondly, and very striking, I think we have a lot of cynicism about the integrity or the values of senior management in our major corporations. Now this is admittedly a skewed sample, but I have found quite the opposite. [I have found] an extraordinarily high level of values, high values, and in fact, sometimes overtly spiritual . . . values. The striking characteristic of these individuals is a strong internal commitment to a set of values.

In some cases these were expressed as explicitly spiritual values, sometimes they were simply that they had a deep commitment to family which they were unwilling to compromise during periods of crisis. Or [they had] a sense of honesty and integrity, personal honesty and integrity. And so under conditions of high stress, they were not about to abdicate that; they were going to stick with their guns. One man at AT&T said, "It's like my compass. When I'm not sure of where I'm going, at least I can look down and it points north." I think that's a wonderful metaphor.

The third dimension [of the three Cs] is control. Now control is not the Machiavellian manipulation of other people. I want to be very, very explicit about that. It's a very particular kind of control which helped me to explain, for the first time in twelve years, research findings we got back in the late 1960s and early 1970s with adept meditators.

Let me give you a very explicit example. This also points to the major transition we're beginning to look at between how the seemingly abstract mental states, points of power and purpose, begin to affect physiology for better or for worse. Control was probably most accurately expressed by a senior manager of Bank of America. He said, "I feel like I'm the director of a play, rather than an actor in it. A director orchestrates and oversees, whereas an actor is sort of pushed around like a puppet—'do this, do that.'" [It is] quite a different perception.

Those people who felt hopeless, who felt helpless, who felt they could not control their destiny, [whether] it was small or large, began to succumb, to get sick and, in fact, to die. One of the things you learn in clinical care is to identify this "helpless, hopeless syndrome." If you have a patient who is doing okay and suddenly they start to look or feel helpless and hopeless, they are going to go into crisis, and if in crisis they are likely going to die.

It's something that sends up a red flag and it did so with these people also. By comparison [there were] those individuals who felt certain. This is not a belief system; this is a certainty that they have that they can influence the course and direction of their lives and the outcome of the reality they choose to develop. Now, fortunately, here it doesn't seem quite so esoteric as it does in some places where I've said this, but it is a volitional reality for them and they did not manifest . . . disease and disability.

This helped me to understand a research finding from over twelve years ago. Because of the early involvement of Ed Mitchell in the founding of Noetic Sciences and their support of our research, we did have access to a number of the early astronauts in our physiology testing program. Now we did one very interesting study which . . . was that we divided [the astronauts] into two groups and they were all given a set of extremely disorienting [conditions]: this room would spin around; they would get loud noises and lights. It was simulating an accident during deep space flight. The two groups were told two different ways of coping with the same set of external problems. One group was told, "Here is a little red button" (actually it was a toggle switch) "and if it gets to be too much, just throw the switch and this problem will stop."

The others were told, "Here is a sequence of things: you have to throw this switch, enter this code, etc., etc. [a difficult complicated task], and that will make this accident abate." Now what they weren't told is that the same accident was happening to . . . [both] groups at the same time. Whether they threw the button or not didn't matter; it wasn't connected. Okay, so this little toggle switch would make absolutely no difference. Now what we counted on was that these macho test pilots would never throw that button because, if they had, the experiment would have been over. And they didn't! No one ever touched that button.

However, the one thing we found is that those individuals (we call them the perceived controlled condition), those astronauts who thought that they could end this by simply throwing that switch [did not show stress]. Their blood pressures did not go up, heart rate did not go up and electrical activity in the brain did not change. In other words, they were not experiencing stress and deterioration changes because they simply believed they were in control. They weren't; they believed that they were. And I really didn't realize what a formidable impact a perceived sense of volitional influence could have until that study and until seeing these executives who seem to have the same quality.

. . . I'll show you just two more [slides] and then we'll have to stop. This dimension of social support sounds rather intangible but, in fact, was the basis of a major campaign in the state of California called Friends Can Be Good Medicine. There is, at this point, unequivocal data that the simple presence of other people [about] whom you care [has a positive effect]. By the way it can even be animals and there's a great research study from Harvard that shows it can even be plants. . . . Someone or something outside of yourself that you feel in interaction with in a meaningful way has a great positive effect.

Men who do not have social support systems, given all other risk factors, have five to six times higher incidence of heart disease. Women who do not have social support systems (all of the factors combined) have three to four times higher incidence of breast cancer. So this, as a factor, in and of itself, is extremely important. So people, to people, are extremely important.

The reason I pictured this at the work place is what we're finding is that whether or not you feel that you can manifest your own belief systems, your own wishes, desires, and direction in the work place is more important than if you can at home. Now we found one ironic finding which is that people who have the lowest social support in the work environment, but the highest social support at home, were the most ill. Now that sounds like a tragic problem. If you think about it, it undercuts the idea that somehow we can go through eight to ten hours of hell in the trenches, come home and everything is fine. It certainly helps [apparently], but it in fact is not real. One of the things we think of is that it's the tea and sympathy syndrome. Instead of helping the person work through the difficulties, it's simply "you're right, they're wrong," and it polarizes the issue into an even more negative set of circumstances.

The very last one I'm going to mention, and I can't show you the details on this, is simply stress management. The point being, every single successful senior manager who made it through times of high stress, had a form of stress management technique. Now for some, it was . . . a meditative practice. Some of them didn't even know it was a meditative practice. We'd ask them, "What do you do?" and they describe this breathing that they do, rhythmic breathing and counting breaths, and I said, "That sounds like Za Sen," and they would say "What?" Or someone would describe this heat rising up in their spinal column and perfusing the brain and giving them an extremely focused and light sense of consciousness, and I'd say it sounds like Kundalini. And they would say "Kundawhat?" The point is that these are not esoteric individuals, they are simply doing it because they learned that it works.

Now one of the last characteristics . . . is . . . that almost all of them have a very particular way of focusing their mind to influence their personal and collective reality. And almost all of them use visualization, in one form or another.

Let me give you an example. At Bechtel Corporation, one of the senior managers (Weinberger and Schultz have come from them; that's the two executives I referred to earlier; they were not part of our study, by the way), this one man said that before the days of computer simulation the reason he rose so rapidly in Bechtel Corporation was because when they were bidding competitively on the structure of a skyscraper, he could visualize; he could see the structure and turn it in space; he could walk inside and go up the elevator shaft, walk the corridors, walk around the building, go up to the top floor, and look down.

It was that skill that enabled him to bid so much more effectively than others who did not have the computer simulation available; the materials, the plan, the bid was always more accurate, and he attributes his success to that major characteristic.

Let's try one ten-second experiential thing. There's no need for preparation. The point is, I think, visualization is made something that is somehow esoteric or abstract or unreal. And I know Martin Rossman is going to give you a very elegant presentation on this. A ten-second visualization is very simply write down the number of windows in your living room on your pad. Could anybody not do that? How did you do it? Think about how you did it. You saw your living room. Right? And you counted the windows- pretty strange! That's visualization. And all of these individuals have some structured way of developing their own visualization techniques.

Now the only place I have never seen this work is [where] I was in the Soviet Union . . . a science city about 200 kilometers east of Moscow. It's a place where they monitor the Soyuz space flights, etc., and a group of us had been invited there to bring a set of very miniaturized biofeedback instruments which the Soviet Union has used on Soyuz flights. [These instruments] were [also] being used on the space shuttle for motion sickness and disorientation.

When I was in the course of teaching there were about 300 Soviet scientists in black suits and white shirts and black ties, sitting in perfect rows. By the way this is a mandatory science city. Scientists from all over the Soviet Union in the biological, medical and space-flight sciences are ordered to come and live there with their families; there are about 23,000 people. It has its own power sources . . . they have their own everything; it's a self-contained city.

So we were discussing this use of biofeedback and instrumentation and the Soviets are quite fascinated by the role of the mind, perhaps in many ways more amenable to the role of mind/body interactions for optimal performance than we are, and they have made better use of it in many ways. We got into the subject of how you control the EEG, how you change the physiological responses and we began talking about visualization. It got sort of abstract and so I said let's try a ten-second visualization. . . .

I said, "Close your eyes and tell me when you can write down on your pads the number of windows in your living room." Immediately, these three hundred scientists just started laughing. Now they never laugh, especially at a presentation like this. Suddenly they just cracked up! My translator (they had these over-sized podiums, so you share the podium with your translator) kind of tugged at my jacket and I turned to him and he said, "Not to worry; they are not laughing at you, the point is that we all live in state housing and everybody has one window in their living room!" And then to add to this, there was one Soviet bilingual scientist in the front row who piped up and said, "Yes, and they are all the same size."

So what I would like to leave you with is that I think that many of the ideas that we are exploring today have very pragmatic [value]. I hopefully have demonstrated that they really have very pragmatic value. They are being used in major corporations, they are part of an ongoing effort in the space program and they are part of an international recognition of the role of mind/body interaction both to define ultimately the nature of the reality in which we find ourselves living and also to modify and change and develop our full potential to states of optimal health and optimal performance. I think it is a quite real effort and we are going to see quite real results from that in the next decade. Thank you.

Chapter Three

IMAGERY IN HEALING

by

Martin Rossman, M.D.

KRISTIE KNUTSON: Ladies and gentlemen, it is my pleasure to introduce to you now our next speaker. Dr. Martin Rossman is the Director and Founder of the Collaborative Medicine Center in Mill Valley, California. He is a Clinical Associate in the Department of Medicine at the University of California Medical Center in San Francisco. He is also in private practice with the use of behavioral medicine and traditional acupuncture. In his lectures and writings, Dr. Rossman has focused extensively on the use of imagery and traditional Chinese acupuncture in the healing process [and the role of imagery] in relaxation and self healing. Indeed, his presentation today will be dealing with imagery and healing. Please join me now in welcoming Dr. Martin Rossman.

MARTIN ROSSMAN: I wanted to start with just one slide in a minute because I always come to these things and I am thinking of what I'm going to say; and then after I listen to speakers like Willis Harman and Ken Pelletier, they stimulate this train of thought and tap different synapses, and [then] different kinds of ways of putting things together start to happen and then I forget about everything I was going to say. . . .

Actually I am here to talk about the imagination in healing and the use of imagery in healing. And I kind of like the way the morning's going with Willis [Harman] talking about global and paradigmatic shifts, about the nature of consciousness and reality, and the implications for us as both individuals and a society, and Ken [Pelletier] kind of bringing it down to specific practical pragmatic uses in the corporate culture which is such an influential portion or segment of our culture.

I'm going to kind of bring it down and share with you some ideas and some ways of using it that I use all the time in my medical practice. I am a general practitioner of medicine. And I've used imagery, or taught imagery to people in my practice for about the last sixteen years. I also enjoy teaching it as a self-care tool, teaching it to health professionals, [and] teaching it to lay people. The title of this seminar is "Mind As Healer"; I think the mind is probably the most widely under-utilized health resource there is. I think there are very few things as powerful as our minds and our attitudes, our beliefs and the way they stimulate our emotions that affect our health and affect our choices.

We don't really know much about it. We don't really even know what it is. I don't think anybody knows what a mind is. But we talk about it, we use it in different ways all the time. And of course there are different faculties of mind that are important in health; will is one, intellect is another, the imagination is another. I think really [imagination] is one of the most important mental faculties that play a part in the development of our health and well-being. I would like to talk about it a little bit. I am not going to spend time, at least much time, on theoretical kinds of matters.

I guess the first thing we ought to talk about is what is imagery and what is an image. The simplest way to think about it, the way I like to think about images is that images are thought forms with sensory qualities. An image is a thought that you can see, or feel, or hear, or smell, or taste, or some kind of combination of those things. Images are internal representations of reality. It's a perfectly normal, natural built-in way that our nervous system (a large part of our nervous system) incorporates, and accesses, and stores information. It's a type of thinking that undoubtedly predates verbal thinking by many tens of thousands of years. If you look back to the cave drawings and so on, and ancient artifactual drawings, you see that people were communicating by the means of images long before written languages ever started to appear. The earliest written languages are picture languages if you look at ancient Chinese and so on. It's just a natural way that we take in the world and represent it to ourselves.

The reason it's important to health is because thoughts are things. Thoughts are real [things] if anything's a thing, and of course now we don't think anything's a thing, as Dr. Harman was saying. We can think of them [thoughts] all as energy, and so we can say that thoughts are energy forms, and that they have tremendous implications in the formation of other energy forms.

The ancient Greeks had—and this is about as far as I'll go theoretically until the end—but the ancient Greeks in the time of Hippocrates had what we would call a psychophysiology. We could call it a metaphysiology that actually is very current and really pretty much forms the basis of the psychoneuroimmunology that Ken [Pelletier] was talking about this morning. And they kind of understood the way the imagination worked. First of all, they considered the imagination as an organ; it was a psychophysiological faculty or organ. It was considered to be as real as your arm or your liver, which of course it is; it's just invisible.

The Greeks said that we apprehended the world, we took in the world, through our senses. We took that [which we apprehended] into our heart, which to them was the seat of the soul, of the psyche [which] lived in the heart, and was the guiding force and guiding principle in life. And there the imagination would form images, would bring together the sensory qualities and leave the matter outside. This was their explanation. They would leave the matter outside and form an image. Now that image, or at least some of the images, would stimulate emotional reactions, positive or negative. It could be either one. But some images would stimulate the emotions. The emotions, in turn, stirred the humors.

You remember the humors. The Greeks had the four humors, melancholic and phlegmatic and so on, and they were believed to be circulating substances or energies that then affected the state of the body. Now if you take the term humors and you substitute the term hormones, and if you include in the class of hormones things like neurotransmitters, and opiate-peptides, and endorphins, and so on and so forth, you really have a very up-to-date kind of model for how we think the imagination works in terms of influencing the body, either negatively or positively.

We have emotional reactions to our belief systems and our thoughts. Those emotions are physical changes, they stimulate physical changes and, of course, all these are mechanisms. But I have found it interesting, in these last ten to fifteen years of paradigmatic shift, to kind of look at these things, and [even] if there wasn't a paradigmatic shift, there are a lot of ways that we can certainly account for many of these phenomena. . . . We know now that the different emotions are psychophysiologic states, and that they are mediated by different brain hormones, and transmitters, and so on and so forth, and [that] they have profound effects in the body.

The most common example of imagery in the way that it works in health, and one that I use a lot to explain it to my patients—I had to bring it down from the airy-fairy realm into the practical—is to talk about worrying. Have you ever worried about anything? Most people have worried about something.

In worrying you sit there and you start thinking about all of the different nasty things that could possibly happen, the doom and gloom and disasters. Whether it's about a big exam, or a job interview, or that you are going to die someday, or nuclear war (or whatever it is) there's plenty around to worry about. If you've never worried, you know, we could probably make you worry and you could experience that.

What you are doing when you are really worried if you have a big event coming up, an exam, an interview, some kind of life crisis that's coming up and you're concerned about what you are going to do, and you are going over and over it in your mind and you're getting tense or you have to run to the bathroom every five minutes or your neck gets real tense, you get a headache, your heart starts pounding fast, your palms are sweating–that's imagery. That's the psychophysiologic power of imagery! You're responding, your body is responding to your thoughts of something that has not happened. It has happened only in your mind and it's happening only as a thought, and as a series of images which is the mediator.

The flip side of that, if we can make ourselves sick that way–and certainly we have learned a lot in the last ten to fifteen years about the physiology of stress and the adverse effects of unrelieved and unmitigated stress on the system so on–but the flip side, is that if we can make ourselves that sick through mental attitudes and through worrying and reacting that way, the potential is there to help make ourselves better and to interrupt that response.

The thing about worrying is that it's the effects of a runaway imagination. It's the effects of an imagination that is not being used on purpose; it's not being used skillfully; it's not being directed. It's running on by habit, and it's running on in reaction and response to all kinds of things that are being fed in. So when you are talking about using imagery for healing there are a number of skills to start to use. [There are] a number of skills to develop that allow you to begin to use your imagination to reverse the effect of worrying to start with, or at least to stop them.

The first imagery skill that I always like to teach people is to stop using imagery. And this is where meditative techniques, [such as] simple relaxation techniques and breathing techniques, whether a mantra or imagining [can help]. Of course, imagery is one of the quickest ways to help people learn to relax and interrupt the ongoing worry response.

If you take a couple of deep breaths, and get yourself comfortable, and let yourself really get into a daydream about being some place that's very beautiful, and very peaceful, and very quiet and relaxed, and really let yourself get into it like you did when you were a kid, you know imagine what you see there, and what you hear, and what you smell, what it feels like to be there and so on and so forth, your body, just like it reacted to the images of doom and gloom, will react to the images of rest and relaxation. Your hypothalamus or your pituitary gland will send the all-clear signal out to your body.

Dr. Irving Oyle who initially introduced me to a lot of things about imagery and visualization years ago makes it very simple. He says, when you focus your mind on images of disasters and catastrophes and so on and so forth, your brain secretes worry juice into your blood. And that's a very accurate way of thinking about it. It's a very simple way to think about the very complex cascade of psycho-physiologic responses that occur in response to stress.

But your brain can also make the antidote to worry juice and when you focus your mind on something that's pleasant, or beautiful, or inspiring, or purposeful, or meaningful, your brain secretes joy juice. There is a physiology of joy, and we're just moving into the area where I think we are about to discover the psychophysiology of joy, of satisfaction, of love, of meaning, and these kinds of things. As Ken showed, challenge, commitment, and control [the three Cs] somehow turn our systems on and make them much more resilient to dealing with the different demands of modern life.

I find this really useful in practice because typically the people that I see in practice are people who are most worried. We get a high incidence of people who are coming in with physical complaints: headaches, or neck aches, or back aches, or heart disease, or high blood pressure, or sexual difficulties, or stomachaches, or colitis, or asthma, or eczema—you know, you can go on and on.

The mind plays a role in all disease and illness. Whether it's responsible one hundred percent or not I'm not even going to get into, but it can play a big role in whether you get better or not. I often see the people who are sort of the best at worrying themselves sick. That can be a very positive thing because, as I say, "Look, your mind has already created some very powerful changes in your body. How would you like to learn to use it in a way that might be able to reverse [these changes] or create some very positive things?

I think it is true that people who tend to respond to worry and stress with physical illness are the people who have the best opportunity to physically change themselves. They are sort of, as Ted Barber refers to them, a group of people who are psychosomatically plastic. In other words, their bodies respond more acutely to the thoughts. And again, if the body is responding to runaway thoughts, random thoughts, scary thoughts, [there is] trouble! If you can start to focus the mind, beginning with relaxation, or focus on something positive or relaxing, you turn off that response and you let the natural healing mechanism of the body begin to work.

Now a great deal of healing begins with relaxation. I just saw an ad last night on television. I don't know how many of you have seen it, but they said, "We asked a thousand doctors if they were stranded on a desert island with only one medication, what would it be?" Have you seen that commercial? I saw it last night. I think the answer was they would take Bayer Aspirin, which isn't a bad choice if it were a medication! But if I were on that island, especially if I had a group of other people that I was caring for there, and if I were somehow limited to only one method of healing somehow (whether a medication, or a procedure, or a technique) and I had to treat everyone who came to see me with just that one technique, it would be with simple relaxation.

I would just teach them how to turn off the stress response because we are the inheritors, we have a birthright, of something like a three and one-half billion-year-old system whose prime desire is to heal itself. It's that built-in homeostatic mechanism that defies our understanding, and it wants to balance, it wants to heal. No matter what's happening, it's doing its best. The system is always doing its best to remain in balance in a rapidly changing world, externally and internally.

Whether you call it the unconscious mind, the inner mind, the psyche, the soul, you know, whatever it is that is alive in us, it is trying to maintain that balance all the time. It knows how to do that far better than our conscious mind can ever comprehend.

So first start with interrupting that stress response and letting your natural healing processes work for you. In self care class we have a set of tapes that teach people sort of one, two, three, here are the steps that we think are most useful. The first step is relaxation. Once you've learned to relax it's obvious, or at least it has been shown, that imagery can have much more specific effects than just simple relaxation on the physiology.

Studies from biofeedback, hypnosis research, [and] imagery research now have shown conclusively that imagery plays a large role in biofeedback, such that even Elmer Green from the Menninger Foundation last year said, "There is no biofeedback, it's all imagery." I guess he should know. He knows a lot more about biofeedback than I know. I was thinking he was selling biofeedback a little short because it helps you tune into the effects of your imagery. But imagery in one way or the other has been shown to affect heart rate, blood pressure, respiratory rate, gastrointestinal motility, gastrointestinal mobility, levels of sexual arousal, EEG patterns, electrical skin responses, levels of muscle tension and immune system responses.

So we see that through imagery we can touch, in effect, all of the major control systems of the body. We're talking about blood flow, we're talking about the circulatory system, the nervous system, and the immune system. These are the major self-regulatory systems of the body and they are all influenced or [are] influenceable by imagery.

Recently there was a study report at the Society for Behavioral Medicine [that will] give you a flavor of how specific the imagery might be. They compared [two] groups of students at one of the colleges in Boston, I think at Harvard, because there's been this controversy in this field [to the effect that]: "Well, are all the effects just due to the relaxation? And visualization and imagery do not really matter [because] it is all the natural healing response."

They were students who had chronic viral infections and recurrent viral infections, so their immune systems weren't working well against viruses.

They taught one group a relaxation technique. They taught the other group a relaxation technique and a visualization, much like a Simonton type visualization where they imagined white blood cells being very aggressive and prolific, and attacking the viruses, and destroying them, and policing the system and so on. What they found was that both the imagery and the imagery plus visualization group had improved; both groups increased the level of salivary IgA, which is an antibody present in the saliva, which represents the body's first line of defense against bacteria and viruses.

Both [groups] raised those [IgA antibodies] equally as compared to a group that was just taught something in educational programs about viruses and so on. But the visualization group, specifically, increased dramatically their circulating levels of what are called helper T4 cells, which are the specific cells that are important in identifying and destroying viral infections, and circulating levels of IgG antibodies, which are antibodies in the blood that were specific against the viruses.

There's been another study from Michigan State University where a group of students were taught to visualize their white blood cells. Neutrophils (one type of white blood cell) circulate through the blood and, when there's an infection or an inflammation, they literally crawl out of the blood vessels, they slip in between the cells of the blood vessels and they migrate into the tissues to the area of infection.

These people were taught to imagine that happening. And they did, and they did! They imagined that happening, and their circulating levels of neutrophils went down. And then they were able to visualize the reverse, and again, the neutrophils seemed to come back into the blood stream. So the specificity of imagery may be much greater than we ever, ever dreamed. I certainly agree with Willis [Harman] and say don't put limits on this because the limits may be much much wider than most people think, if there are limits. (I'm sort of a believer in limits myself; [that] may be my limitation, [in fact] I'm sure that's my limitation; I feel more comfortable somehow with limits.)

Certainly when it comes to influencing our health for better or for worse, we have much, much more control then most of us give ourselves credit for. Some people think we have ultimate control, that it is all up to us, and it may be. Even if you don't believe that, there is a tremendous way to go before you even have to deal with that one.

There is something that to me is more profound and interesting about imagery than what I call directive imagery, or programming imagery which is this idea of [saying] "Okay, now I'm going to sit down, I'll relax, I'll focus my mind, and I'm sort of going to direct my unconscious mind to create these positive changes in my body." And of course this can be a great thing to do, this relaxation or pain relief.

We know people can have major operations under hypnosis which is basic hypnosis imagery. That's imagery in a relaxed state of mind, most of it. We know people are capable of doing these remarkable things as Ken Pelletier shared with you: sticking knitting needles through their arms, and increasing their heart rate to three hundred [beats] a minute, and reducing it again. [There are] people who are adept at these things. But I think that even more important than the fact that imagery is a way we can focus our intention and tell our unconscious mind what to do, is the fact that imagery is a natural language of the unconscious mind, and that we can learn through our imagery from our unconscious mind what to do.

The idea of a twenty-seven-year-old, a thirty-five-year-old, a sixty-five-year-old conscious mind telling a three and one-half billion-year-old unconscious mind what to do in this situation, is sort of patently absurd. It ignores the idea which is really fundamental. I learned this from traditional Chinese medicine. Then I learned more and more about traditional medicines, as Ken [Pelletier] said, and learned that our present state of medicine is a deviation (sort of an exploration into something new) but really is different than any other medicine that has ever been on the face of the earth.

[In traditional medicines] a symptom is regarded as feedback. A symptom is not something to be obliterated. A symptom is something that is calling for your attention. And even in Western medicine we acknowledge that. The only difference is that we usually say that it is telling you to go see your doctor, or that it needs some Valium, or that it needs Bayer Aspirin. That doesn't mean that those things are not all useful, but a symptom is a very personal message, and it's much like the usual analogy that we draw, that it's like the oil light in your car. You wouldn't, if you were driving down the freeway, and the oil light in your car came on, you wouldn't pull it into the gas station and ask the mechanic to tape it over because it was making you nervous, and was interfering with your life. Nobody would do that!

"I am very busy, and I have a full schedule, and everything is planned out for the next eighteen years, and you know, the light makes me anxious, so could you pull the wires out or tape it over?" That's want we're asking our doctors to do; and that's what we're teaching our doctors to do also. This is not the doctors' fault; this comes from the culture because we want a quick fix, an easy answer to what are often complex solutions. And there is nothing wrong with that except it doesn't work. It's not a moral issue, it just doesn't work.

We look at a symptom as something that is calling for our attention and then the question is, What is it saying to us? Once we get to the place, "Okay, I'm willing to pay attention," how do we get to what it's saying? Here imagery really shines. Imagery is the natural language of the inner mind or the unconscious. I like the way that Ira Progoff said it. He is a depth psychologist, a Jungian, and he says that (and it's a beautiful quote): "Movement in the depths of being is the way the psyche carries out its directive role in man." He used the psyche (the psyche of course means soul) as the guiding principle: whatever it is that is alive in us, whatever it is that has lived through all the different bodies you had in this life—not even talking about past lives. You know, you've had a billion bodies in this life. You don't have the same body you had at five, or twelve, or twenty-four, or even yesterday actually; the body is always changing.

There is something in there that hasn't changed much since you've started to become aware of it [since you were] three, four, five years old. There is something behind all of our eyes that hasn't changed a whole lot, no matter how many bodies we've been through. He calls it the psyche, and he says it's the guiding principle, and that it moves at deep levels of being, and that's how it performs its directive role; and that the content of that movement is imagery. So that by tuning in to our internal imagery, [we are tuning in to] a natural language of the psyche, of the unconscious, of the soul as it were. I sometimes tell people this. I talk to people, to my patients, and tell them to think about this: there is something in you that has guided your development from a single microscopic cell in your mother's ovary to whatever you are now. It got you from a single cell to two cells, four cells, eight cells, the whole process up to getting little baby you, and then you kept changing very, very rapidly, and [then there was] five-year-old you, and twelve-year-old you, and twenty year old you, and so on and so forth.

There is something whether you call it unconscious mind, psyche, soul, DNA, genes, God, Jesus, whatever it is, there's something in you that knows how to do this. Otherwise we would just be mudpuddles. If you put us in a blender, that's what we would come out as. We are mudpuddles, about sixty-five, seventy percent water and a bunch of chemicals. But something in us is getting that mudpuddle to grow arms and legs, and think, and do things, and so on and so forth. So something is organizing this matter-energy into very unlikely forms, statistically unlikely forms, such as individual human beings.

There is a part of all of us that knows how to do that. It creates your body, and recreates your body, and recreates your body. You know, there is a common sense misunderstanding about the body. We think of bodies as things. Bodies are not things. They are more accurately processes, flows of energy. And that's not a mystical idea, that's just a physiologic reality even in Western physiology. A cell is a living thing; it's constantly changing; it's taking in nutrients; it's rebuilding its worn out parts; it's getting rid of waste products so it's not the same cell it was even a few minutes ago. And yet it has an identifiable form. It's like the old Zen saying about how you can't step in the same river twice. So the river has a form, but the stuff is changing, and that's what our bodies are like.

There's some part of you that is keeping it together in a reasonably identifiable, coherent kind of form. So there's something in you that is intelligent enough to make your body in the first place from nothing; if you'll grant that and then say, "Well, maybe if it's intelligent enough to make my body and my head, maybe it could make me a headache, if it wanted to tell me something. If it could make my head, it could probably make a headache." That's logical. "If it's making a headache and it's making a headache for a reason (to try to get me to pay attention to something) it makes sense that, if I got quiet and listened and looked, it would tell me why."

It's easier to make a thought or an image than it is to make a headache. And certainly much easier than to make a head. So you're talking about energy-efficient forms of communication. And what we need to do is to get quiet enough to listen. We need to reown our respect for life, our respect for our own lives. There is something happening in our lives, whether we know what it's doing or not, that seems to be doing something, seems to have a purpose. It's capable of incredibly complex systems of organization.

To get quiet enough to listen is, of course, the perennial wisdom. [It is] to listen to that inner guidance, the still silent voice within.

An illness is a form of inner guidance. My colleague and good friend Dr. Naomi Remen, who works a lot with imagery and works a lot with people with serious illnesses, has an interesting concept. She says "It's possible that illness, that serious illness, may be a Western form of meditation." And you see this in medicine all the time. It's that people don't stop; they don't stop and listen, and re-evaluate, and take life seriously very often until there's a major crisis.

That crisis is often a health crisis. It's at those times in your life when you stop and you look around and say "What am I doing? Do I want to keep doing it that way, or do I want to change? Please God, if you let me survive this . . . if I survive this heart attack, I'll do this, that, the other thing." And people make big life changes after their heart attacks, or when they develop cancer, when they develop serious illnesses.

Now it would be nice to [make the life changes] before that [crisis] had to happen. And a lot of what Ken was talking about, of course, in the usefulness of quieting, regular listening within, regularly paying attention, or listening to the symptoms earlier, many people have found—I know Ken has done some research on this, and I certainly found it, and many other people have found it—that if you take somebody with a serious illness and you go back, taking a careful history, you will find out they were getting messages for a long time. It doesn't come out of the blue. I think one of our big cultural fears is that "Oh God, this cancer, it just comes out of the blue. It's like an evil spirit. It's like a disincarnate entity which just sort of roams around, picks you, and comes down." I don't think that's true.

People were getting symptoms and signals long before, and coping with them, or stuffing them behind [in the back of their minds], and not listening. This doesn't mean you should live in fear of your symptoms, but [you should] take some time to listen to your body. Your body will transmit messages of your emotions, of your spirit, of your soul, and of your mind if that's the way it can get your attention.

So we use a couple of different techniques which we teach in our self-care series, the "Imagine Health" series, and I use them in my practice all the time. One is just having people tune in to the symptom itself, getting quiet, and allowing an image to form for the symptom, and [then] examining and observing [the image]. Then we even get people talking to it [the image], and letting it talk back to them. We engage in this inner dialogue, "Why are you here? What do you want from me? What do you have to offer me if I give you what you want?"

Start to work with this as a meaningful event and one that doesn't necessarily mean you harm. Let me give you a quick example. Simple visualization is sometimes enough, but often it leads to a much deeper appreciation of yourself as a whole person. A young man about twenty-six, very successful, is an executive manager who had a serious connective tissue disease which is one of the ninety-five percent of all illnesses for which we don't know the cause, nor do we know the cure. He also had recurrent ulcers, peptic ulcers, stomach ulcers.

I was working with him for a while and he started to redevelop an ulcer. We started to work on his major disease, and as he started to get close to [the cause] he started to get very anxious, and sure enough, he started to redevelop an ulcer. So I had him focus on the pain in the stomach, the ulcer pain, to get an image for that. An image that came to mind was a little fire burning there. And he said, "Yeah, it feels hot and there's a fire burning there." I said, "Well, maybe there's something that you could do to help make it feel better."

He played around a little while, and imagined running cool, blue water through it. He saw it putting out the fire, then he opened his eyes and said, "I can't believe it, it feels better!" And he was so excited to find that there was something he could do to make his stomach pain feel better. He was really enthused about it. He went home, and for about the next two or three weeks he said, "Anytime I feel anything in my stomach I run this water through it and it goes away." And he was real happy with that.

He comes back in [the office] a few weeks later and his stomach pain is back! No matter how much imaginary cold water he runs through, he can't relieve the pain. So I said, "Well, let's see what's going on now." This time he focuses in, he gets a hand that's pinching. He says he sees it pinching his inside. I said, "Well, who's on the other end of the hand?" He couldn't see that, [so] we explored the hand a little bit with some things we usually do. And I said, "Well, just ask the hand why it's pinching you." And he said it let go of his stomach and it started shaking at him like that [threateningly]. And he said, "It's really angry at me." I said, "Ask the hand why it's angry at you, and give the hand a voice and let it answer you. This is all imaginary but just sort of suspend your judgment for awhile." And he said, "It's going like this [beckoningly]. It wants me to come with it." And I said, "Well, are you willing to go with [it]?" He said, "Yes." And so he goes with it, and the hand goes like this [pointing], it points to this bag. He says, "There's this bag. It's sort of a pinkish white bag, and it's like there's a bunch of things in there and they are all pushing and poking to get out, and stretching the bag." Then I said, "Well, can you see in the bag?" and he said, "No I can't."

So I said, "Well, imagine that you can see through the bag." So he starts and says "Oh!" And I said, "What's happening?" And he says, "You know," and he starts crying.

After he's done crying, which took awhile, he said, "My heart is in that bag. And there are all kinds of sharp things, zooming around, and all kinds of dangerous things in there that are bouncing off the walls, and they keep bumping and bruising my heart." And so I asked him, "What do you want to do?" And he said, "Well, I've got to get it out of there somehow." And I asked him, "How are you going to do it?" And he said, "I don't know." So I said, "Ask the hand if it has some advice for you." And the hand told him to untie the bag, and imagine taking out one thing at a time. This imaginary hand told him that! It said, "It's too much, you can't open the bag all at once. Open the bag and I'll take out one thing at a time for you to look at." And he said, "Okay," and the hand reaches in the bag, and it comes out, and he sees his stepfather.

He gets into a whole thing, he starts crying, he gets angry about how he resented his stepfather when he came into his house. And there's about two or three sessions on real rage that he felt within him, getting into how he felt with his mother, and how he got [along] with his real father, and how he felt with his stepfather . . . and the whole thing . . . what he got out of it was that he always stuffs his emotions; he eats his emotions, and he holds them in this bag, and he had been holding them in for a long time, and this was damaging his heart, his vitality and it would go out into the different organs.

It really clicked with him. He had thought, sort of on the outside for awhile, that he was holding this inside but never really got the connection with his physical health. And over a process that took about nine months with him, he was able to use that imagery process to take out these things, one by one, to deal with them, and to come to terms with his emotions, and feel better right in proportion with how he worked through his feelings. With some people it's much shorter and with some it's longer. He has a serious chronic illness that's of something like fourteen years duration, so nine months of work is actually pretty quick. He learned how to use that [process] so that the guidance that's in there, that can come through illness and symptoms is, I think, one of the most profound uses of imagery.

We use other techniques, like a talk with an imaginary wise figure, or an inner advisor (we call it an inner guide) to imagine you're in a beautiful place with a wise loving figure that knows you very well, and to have a talk with it about what's going on just like it was really there. This is one of the very, very profound and useful techniques for people.

I think the key is to take these things, take symptoms and illnesses, consider that they might be meaningful, that they might actually mean you no harm, that there may be something to learn from them, and appeal to your inner mind. Get quiet, and ask for help, and pay attention. As Willis said, when you ask for help, it's something like praying; it's very similar to the real process of praying. And you'll be surprised that it [help] will often be there. So thank you for your attention and I'm looking forward to the rest of the day along with the rest of you.

Chapter Four

GENERAL DISCUSSION I

with

Drs. Harman, Pelletier, Rossman, Brauer, and Wilson

ONSLOW WILSON: I've been keeping notes because I know there's going to be an exam after this, you see. There's going to be a test, and if any of you think you're going to get out of here without passing this test, you can forget it. As you are well aware, this is a museum, and if you check the basement, you will see we have some mummies down there. Those are the ones who did not pass the test. They never left. [laughter]

I want to start with the business of multiple personalities that Dr. Harman mentioned in his talk this morning. I found that to be particularly exciting, and I wondered if you [Dr. Harman] could elaborate a little more on that while we wait for some questions to come our way.

WILLIS HARMAN: The only part you really need for the examination is the question, Can we expand on the idea of multiple personalities? I didn't pay him to ask that, but actually the most exciting thing to me about the multiple personalities is that in some recent work it turns out that although these personalities are all very different, (most of them seem to have originated in early childhood due to extreme sexual or physical abuse) . . . there is often one that is a healer, that really knows how to heal. And you can talk to that one, and get some advice, and also it takes care of emergencies, like healing third degree burns overnight and things like that.

But the particularly exciting thing about the multiples to me is that one of these multiple [personalities] seems to be unique in that it answers questions like, When did you come into being? and that kind of question—it answers them quite differently. This particular one is always very cooperative, and very positive in terms of its emotional response. In fact, they sometimes call it the Inner Self Helper. When this one is asked "When did you come into being?" it answers something like, "I have always been." And when it is asked about death, it says, "Well, all the other personalities disintegrate and the physical body decays, but I remain." So you can see it's a neat little window into some fundamental mystery that we can use for some research work. It's got the scientists pretty puzzled.

ALAN BRAUER: I would like to make a comment about that. I'm interested in multiple personalities also for a couple of practical reasons in that I have several patients who are multiples. One of them probably will win some kind of an award because she had, at the time I first started to see her, thirty-two different personalities. I took this as a challenge. I can report that she now has forty-one. So I'm not sure that we're heading exactly in the right therapeutic direction.

However, there's certainly a lot of questions as to whether or not multiple personalities is really a legitimate syndrome. Many therapists feel that it's really just a person's imagination or it's acting. I have rather an open mind about that. I think that if a person feels that he has a certain number of personalities and appears to act differently in different situations, then you have to accept that as being real, which is what I've done, particularly with this "multiple-multiple." What's happening, though, although she's getting more personalities, is that they're getting less distinct. And she's having much more difficulty calling up a particular one, which leads me to think that something real is happening. She is, in a sense, becoming more integrated. I suppose if we go to larger and larger numbers of personalities, she'll be just like the rest of us. Because we are all different people at different moments—it's like the river that's always different. We're all different at every given instant. So possibly we should head in the direction (therapeutically) with this person, and maybe with other multiples, of allowing them as much variation as possible, and discussing what it means to be in a particular frame, and why that has come up at this particular moment.

ONSLOW WILSON: That's very interesting, because it says to me that if I were to drag out one of my personalities at this time, one who likes to behave in certain ways that would affect my physiology in a way that would manifest diabetes, for example, I would show all of the symptoms of a diabetic right now. Is that correct? Is that not what we're saying?

KENNETH PELLETIER: That is what Dr. Harman was reporting, and that's really fascinating.

WILLIS HARMAN: It takes a little while, I think.

KENNETH PELLETIER: Let me respond to that. Actually there are two factors that have been documented in the literature which would mediate against simple acting. One is that the shift between diabetic positive and diabetic negative is quite rapid—within a matter of minutes. The other is that when you follow the EEG tracings, which are fairly stable, at least in the short run, they change over time; as we age, our EEG changes. But for relatively stable periods of time—years—it stays as distinct as our fingerprints. And yet, when you have a multiple personality, the electroencephalogram between one and the other [personality] is as distinct as between any two people. To me, that part of the multiple personality work is fascinating because it does begin to look like, in a somewhat uncontrolled fashion, precisely the same thing we saw on the adept meditators many years ago, which is that certain mental states then have a profound influence on subsequent physical functions.   And again, it mediates somewhat against [the idea] that this is a purely illusory phenomenon.

ONSLOW WILSON: Okay, I want you to keep talking, Kenneth, because I have a question for you. "Dr. Pelletier, what can you tell us about homeopathy?"

KENNETH PELLETIER: Probably very little.   Homeopathy, as you know, is clearly not an area in which I have expertise, although I find it to be of interest.   George Vithoulkas, who is probably the most eminent homeopath in the world at this point in time, has trained and worked with a group of physicians in Berkeley, allopathically trained physicians. . . . Roger Morrison, in particular, who heads the Hahnemann Medical Clinic in Berkeley has, each fall, an ongoing seminar where George Vithoulkas teaches. Now although we don't, within our division of Internal Medicine, have homeopathy as a service yet, what I have found is a willingness at least to refer people to, in particular, this homeopathic group in Berkeley, and again, it's rather like the executives in these corporations.   The result is sometimes very dramatic with conditions that do not improve by virtue of an allopathic intervention, and sometimes do not improve by way of psychological intervention.

Now the question in my mind is that everything that we know, beyond a certain dilution of the homeopathic remedy, then goes quite rapidly beyond (quote) Avogadro's number, which is [to say] that the molecular constituent [of the active substance] suddenly disappears.   There's literally no molecule of the original substance left, and yet, at these increasingly high dilutions they [homeopaths] do report therapeutic benefit.   To me that's interesting because the best homeopaths I've ever seen work, work in a way that, to me, is strikingly similar to how Marty [Dr. Rossman] works, which is they take psychological factors into account. There's a tremendous placebo enhancing response in the kind of detailed history and care that a good homeopathic physician gives. . . . They state this quite openly; the administration of the homeopathic substance often will elicit either a mental image or a physiological state that recalls some previous trauma that bears on the disease. So in a sense, perhaps homeopathy then becomes one of a number of approaches in a total patient care approach. Certainly it deserves more merit than it's given. But again, I don't think the practitioners themselves often know what part [the homeopathic substance] plays. And we need, again, a dialogue.

ALAN BRAUER: A thought occurs to me: I wonder if one of the reasons for the success of homeopathy has to do with the fact that because the doses are so low, and the effects are subtle, the individual is forced to put additional attention on his body, or on the symptom.

KENNETH PELLETIER: Interesting! Very, very likely! It seems consistent with their work.

ONSLOW WILSON: I've got a comment that I'd like to add to that. I read a book recently in French called, in English, *The Alchemy of Life.* In that book, there is reference to the various forms of water; water can exist in many aggregate forms, as we know. [According to the author] one of these forms, which is a form in which there are three molecules of water involved, somehow stimulates the physiology for some reason or another. And I wonder if this business of homeopathy, where you are diluting beyond, as you [Dr. Pelletier] said, Avogadro's number, where there is no molecule [of the active ingredient] left in there—you can make those calculations—I'm wondering if this dilution process is not a process whereby we're altering the configuration, or the ratio of the configuration, of water molecules one with the other.

KENNETH PELLETIER: Actually this harkens back to a project that the Institute of Noetic Sciences supported for a period of time where a group, including the physicist Hal Puthoff from Stanford Research Institute, an immunologist, myself, and Roger Morrison, the homeopathic physician I mentioned earlier, met on a regular basis to try to think through the nature of subtle energy interactions that would then influence something as gross and material as the body.

One of the things that Hal Puthoff pointed out—and I can't repeat this because he's a brilliant physicist—but he did point out that beyond a certain level of dilution, because there is no therapeutic efficacy reported . . . (in terms of how a physicist would view this) it would seem to indicate that there is transmission of information. And that beyond a certain point that information is distorted to the point where it's no longer communicating anything. There is some research that has come out of London that the reconfiguration of the water molecule, the hydrogen oxygen complex . . . is a finite number—and by some calculations he [Hal Puthoff] did, it would correspond with the finite number of dilutions in which you have therapeutic efficacy. There is a finite number of configurations in which this molecule could be bent, and at the "bend" of a molecule is information. Perhaps one of the ways in which the dilution is acting is [by] communicating the original information from the substance in the form of a molecular twist or reconfiguration. That's about as far as it went, but at least that was some of the speculation.

ALAN BRAUER: I want to point out when we're talking about low doses in activity, that one of the most active mind substances comes in millionths of a gram, and that's LSD. And just think of the incredibly potent effects of that level of dose, which is much smaller than any other psychoactive drug that we use.

ONSLOW WILSON: I think I can hear my boss saying, "Look, these guys are getting too technical," so I'm going to switch. You [Dr. Rossman] haven't said very much since we have been up here, so I have a question for you. Dr. Rossman, "Can an incurable disease, like Parkinson's Disease, be cured by imagery?"

MARTIN ROSSMAN: I'm going to answer that two different ways. One, I think that that's possible. You know when we are talking about curing illnesses through imagery and through mental means, you've got some really interesting phenomena that have yet to be accounted for. For one thing, it seems like everybody who ever seriously looked at the effects of the mind on the body agrees that the lowest common, or highest common, denominator is belief.

This goes through homeopathy, it goes through acupuncture, it goes through Western medicine, it goes through surgery, it goes through biofeedback, it goes through religion; it may be that the most potent healer is what you believe will heal you. The way that impacts on whether or not "incurable" diseases, like Parkinson's, can be cured is that if a person—and we don't know the limits of this—if a person really believes, and has the support, and is working the right way, I think that there's definite hope for any illness . . . [there are] people [who] have . . . spontaneous remission. They have recovered from just about every known reported illness to the surprise of their doctors.

Parkinson's is an illness, specifically, that can take a variety of different courses, often characterized by exacerbations or flares and remissions. I always thought that Parkinson's was sort of a hard-wired disease. When I got my first patient who came to me for acupuncture and imagery for Parkinson's, I called up his neurologist. And I said, "Well, look, this person is here,"—this was a while ago and I was sort of shuffling my feet—"and wants to sort of try some different things, and I haven't seen anybody with this before, and is that okay?" I was basically asking him if it was okay with him, and would he keep seeing the patient, even though [the patient] was obviously crazy, and

I was, too. And he said, "Well, it's probably not going to hurt him and you may get a placebo effect." And I said, "Oh, I didn't know placebo effect worked in Parkinson's disease," and he said, "Oh yeah! You walk into a room full of people with Parkinson's disease,"—which is characterized by a slowness of movement and difficulty starting and stopping—he says, "Walk into a conference room with people with Parkinson's disease and yell, 'Fire!' and you'll have an empty room in no time."

That isn't to diminish the importance of it [the disease] or the severity of it, and so on and so forth, but what he was pointing out was that there was a known, very active placebo effect in Parkinson's Disease, like in many other diseases. This is one of the things that confounds the research that's going on in medications, because many, many medications work initially with Parkinson's and then they stop. [This] is attributed to the placebo effect which always brings up that question: What's happening? Why can someone get better because they have hope, and because there is a new medication and they take it? Then later on it pans out that it [the medication] doesn't have the physical effect that is [in any way] helpful. But those people were better for three weeks, or three months. What is that? And how can we touch it? And I think that we can learn to touch it, [although] we haven't yet.

The other aspect of imagery and belief in healing that's important is that belief is a very fragile thing in some circumstances. And as your culture believes, as your family believes, as your friends believe, as your doctors believe, all these things have powerful [effects]. People now who are trying to work with serious illnesses with imagery and visualization are swimming against—I think the current has reversed—but they're swimming against a tremendous amount of indoctrination and cultural belief and people who say, "No" and people who say, "You're off the wall," and "That's not going to help; well, it won't hurt you," but they don't give it any credit, and that makes it harder.

[But] I think when we get to the place where people realize the tremendous healing potential of the mind, and take it for granted—when everyone realizes that you can help yourself get better from a sore throat more quickly with imagery, the same way we think of a shot of penicillin—when this is kind of taken for granted, it's no issue, it's no big deal. [When all this happens] it's going to be much easier for people to work on all kinds of things with imagery. There's going to be a ripple effect that's going to empower people, and it's going to kind of grow exponentially. That's what I think is going to happen. I think the possibility is there. The way to find out is to learn how to do it, get some good guidance, and do it! Work hard on it for a finite period of time, three weeks, three months, see where you are. That's how you'll find out.

KENNETH PELLETIER: You know, [two] things were triggered [for me] about this malleability, or the change-ability of the supposed hard-wired, organic disease by mental imagery. One is a clinical observation, the other is a study. Clinically . . . if we try a visualization technique . . . we say . . . "Initially the results are imaginary because when you start to say, 'I want my right index finger to increase in temperature,' it is an illusion." But what we have found clinically is that as you repeat that, as you, in fact, establish this communication, it is often through imagery that the physiological change actually begins to happen. And at the point at which the actual physiology follows the image or the verbal command, that's when you begin to get a decline of symptoms. We've actually seen this . . . [that as] the direct ability to influence some physical function increased on the objective basis, you find that symptoms began to fall off.

I was really struck by your talking about the specificity of visual imagery [because of] one of the studies that we have just completed in the area of psychoneuroimmunology. We looked at chronic asthmatics. We did three interventions with groups of asthmatics. One was a relaxation only. The other was a relaxation plus a very general imagery, where they were to just see themselves outdoors and feeling relaxed, with their lungs breathing easily. The third was where they actually were instructed to go inside their lungs and to focus on the mast cells which mediate between the immune response and anything that comes into the lungs. . . .

What we found after three months of intervention was that the people [for whom it] had the least amount of effectiveness, although it [had some], . . . were the relaxation-only group. On the other hand, the people who had the most efficacy were those who had the relaxation plus the specific visualization to their lungs, and the [remaining] group struck somewhere in between. Now that's very convincing evidence because the standard pharmacological model is dose response. When you give "X" amount, you get this much response. When you give "X" more, you get that much more response, and so on, until you hit some toxicity level. And the fact that you can start demonstrating dose response through imagery, with its resulting effect on the physical body, is a line of evidence that's very powerful, or line of inquiry in research that is very powerful.

ONSLOW WILSON: I have another question for you, Dr. Rossman. It's a follow-up, really. "Have you used this method [of imagery] successfully with borderline patients?"

MARTIN ROSSMAN: I was hoping you were going to skip this one, only because it's very complicated. The short answer is yes and no; it depends. You know, imagery is a way of thinking, so in a way we're always using imagery. If somebody comes into my office and tells me their story, and they say, "What do you think I've got, what do you think I should do, and what will happen?" I just tell them [the answers to their questions] and we don't do any relaxation, we don't do any visualization, and so on and so forth. I believe that's a form of imagery, that my words are translated into their inner perceptions of what is likely to happen.

All psychotherapy, even if it seems to be verbal, makes use of imagery as well. The borderline patients—and I assume that you mean patients who "have somebody home," where there's sort of a central being who can either identify or dis-identify with the illness—I think that imagery is most successful with people who "have somebody home." I think it [imagery] is more potent there. But I have worked with some people who seem to be [what] I would call "borderline-borderline." The psychotherapy of borderline patients is a very long, drawn-out affair, and it requires a lot of support and a lot of just relationship in being there.

In the course of that we may use imagery at different junctions to help people start to develop some sense of self. I've done it a couple of times. It's something that I don't do a lot of; I usually refer those people to psycho-therapists, some of whom use imagery, and some who don't.

ONSLOW WILSON: This question has to be a question from a Rosicrucian. I don't know which one of you wants to answer it, but the question is: "Which body becomes ill first? The psychic body or the physical body?" I think, translated into common parlance, the question really is: Does the mind become ill first and the body follow?

WILLIS HARMAN: I'm not sure how meaningful the question is actually, since these things are all part of the same system. But to whatever extent it is meaningful, then the answer is partly a matter of the assumptions that you start from, I think. I was contrasting, when I was speaking earlier, two fundamental views of the universe. The current scientific one which says that matter-energy is real, and mind is derivative in some sense. And then the one that I think we're moving toward, in science as well as outside, which says that the fundamental stuff of the universe is consciousness, and matter-energy is derivative. Now you don't prove one set of metaphysical principles is right and another one is wrong. What you do is live by one and see how it works out. And we've been living by one that's not working out very well, so we're shifting to another one which will probably work out better, and in that other one you are going to put consciousness first.

ONSLOW WILSON: Keep talking, Willis, because the next question is really yours. "Can you begin to outline the main principles of a paradigm that could form the framework of thinking and working and teaching?"

WILLIS HARMAN: I think that it's a very worthy project and it's worth starting on, and we are going to start on it, and we have in a way; it's probably a pretty big project, too. I think you can imagine that chemistry and physics aren't going to change too much when you shift the assumptions underlying them. I think you can imagine that evolutionary theory and psychology are going to change a whole lot, and the training of executives is already changing, and we'll get this into the schools eventually, but that probably won't be early in the game.

MARTIN ROSSMAN: There are some nice things happening in the schools, just on a real simple level—they are not on global levels—but my three-year-old daughter goes to a preschool now. And they taught her how to relax. They aren't teaching her metaphysics yet, but they taught her how to relax. They said, "Make your arm real tense, and now let it go floppy." And now at three-and-a-half she knows how to relax her whole body. My practice consists (yours [Dr. Brauer] probably does too, and I know Ken's does) of just teaching endless numbers of people how to breathe, and how to relax their bodies, at least as starting places.

WILLIS HARMAN: I just don't want it to be misunderstood. I think there are some wonderful things happening with individual teachers behind closed classroom doors, and in some private schools. I really had in mind the school system . . . it's a conservative organization by definition. It's conserving the wisdom of the past, and bringing it forward. It's probably one of the last institutions to change in any major social movement. It sounds contradictory that some of the most exciting things are happening in education in one sense, and the institution is lagging in another sense.

ONSLOW WILSON: The next question is: "Are you aware of any significant influence of color, so that we should wear one color and avoid another?"

MARTIN ROSSMAN: I'm going to start back a little bit . . . I think colors are significant to people in many ways. Colors are certainly personally significant. Colors have emotional meanings to people, and depending on their backgrounds, their metaphysical backgrounds, their philosophical backgrounds, people have very deep beliefs about color—even people who are not involved overtly in metaphysical kinds of practices.

In traditional Chinese medicine, color is used as a diagnostic clue . . . because that system of medicine attempts to look at the energy status of the body. The Chinese said that the universe was energy. . . . There's a book that's five thousand years old that says that. So we try and look, through a traditional diagnosis, at people physically, emotionally, mentally, spiritually—there's a whole system of correspondences, one of which is color. Do you have any favorite colors? Are there any colors that you don't like? Certainly diagnostically, emotionally, [color is important], and I find a real use in asking people what colors mean to them, and I watch what [colors] they are wearing. We use it all the time in terms of diagnosis. . . .

Then there are the actual physical effects of colors, and colors, of course, are vibrating energy at different frequencies. I don't have any doubt that they have effects, [although] I'm not sure what they are. Different traditions attribute different [effects]. The one I like is healing, the color of healing. [From my point of view], every color is a color of healing. [Some people] say, "Green, that's the color of healing!" And then [others say], "Blue, that's healing"; or, "Purple—oh, what does that mean to you?" "Oh, that's the color of healing." In one way or another, they are all the color of healing.

ALAN BRAUER: A couple of years ago the Santa Clara County Jail did an experiment. They painted cells different colors, and looked at (in a not perfectly scientific way, as you can imagine in the penal system) the mood effects, the behavioral effects on the occupants of those cells, and they found that color seemed to make a difference, although not quite in the way that the people had expected. The color that seemed to be the most quieting, at least as reported in the Journal of the Mercury News [a San Jose daily newspaper], was a pastel pink that actually had the calmest effect. You can do with that what you want, go home and paint your walls pink, if you dare.

KENNETH PELLETIER: That's the color of healing!

ALAN BRAUER: Possibly! I can also recall during my internship at Bellevue Hospital [New York City], Bellevue was decorated by someone who thought, probably forty or fifty years ago, that it would be nice to cheer up the inmates, so it looked like a rainbow. Different parts of the walls were painted in different colors—violent green and orange and purple. It was really bizarre. I mean it looked like a patient had decided he was going to use his creative genius. And there were a lot of observations, and even some complaints.

It just happened that the year that I was there they repainted, at least the ward that I was stationed on, a neutral kind of beige. It was certainly more pleasing to me, and to those of us working there, and it seemed to have (again not scientifically) a more calming effect on the patients as well. It was hard to tell, but certainly there was less talk about the colors on the wall. So I suspect that these kinds of things do have more importance than what we really have looked at, and I am intrigued that with the panel of experts here, none of us can really think of any organized studies to investigate this.

ONSLOW WILSON: Perhaps the influence on the patients came from you, because you felt better about the color. There's a question here directed to the panel. "I work with patients who have experienced a death of a child by miscarriage, stillbirth, or newborn death. What do you feel is the impact of the mother's mind on the development of the unborn child?"

KENNETH PELLETIER: One of the most articulate people I've heard turns out, perhaps fortunately, unlike the panel, not to have any degrees that he feels he has to defend. [He is] Joseph Chilton Pearce in *Magical Child.* I think that book is the best articulated statement I've seen of both the somewhat esoteric views and the hard science views of both pre-birth and immediately postpartum [influences] on the infant. I think the minimum you could say scientifically is that the mother's mood changes her body's chemistry. There's absolutely no question about that. And the fact is, the fetus is, until the umbilical cord is severed, an organ of the mother; they're inextricable.

. . . It's known that, for instance, mothers will tell you that if they drink caffeine, about fifteen minutes later, which would be the right assimilation period, the fetus will start to kick. There's no doubt about the fact that the mother and child are inextricably bound during the prepartum state certainly, and afterwards. Again if you look to just the orthodox scientific literature—Jean Piaget's in France, on the developmental stages which Pearce does work with in the course of the book, *Magical Child*—very clearly the early infantile learning, concrete learning, how the brain begins to hard-wire and circuit itself, is profoundly influenced by the mother, and the mother only.

This is what they call [the] bonding process.   So it's clearly a powerful influence, both physically and mentally, if not spiritually.

MARTIN ROSSMAN: I hear a concern in that question about, you know, did the mother cause that [the stillbirth, or death of a newborn child, or miscarriage]—is the mother responsible for that?   And I think what is probably, clinically, a more important question is, What is the effect of the stillbirth, or death of a newborn child, or miscarriage, on the mother's mind?   The mother is the one who's still here, that we can deal with, and I think we really don't know whether or not we're responsible for things like that [death].   We all have a philosophy, and we live by that, and die by that.

But where responsibility comes in, and that is unquestioned, is what you do from that point on.   One of the ways, one of the very powerful uses of imagery that I've used a great deal during that last fifteen years, is in working with people who are grieving.

The first experience was with a woman who had lost a child, and felt very guilty about it, and wondered if she caused that, and if she was responsible, since she was responsible for everything.   And we did an intervention at the time—it just sort of came.   I asked her to get an image for the child, and she imagined the fetus.   It was a miscarriage, an advanced miscarriage, and I asked her to have a talk with it and describe it.   She said it was a boy, and it looked healthy and it was happy.   And I said, "Ask it how it's doing."   And the image said back to her that it was doing fine.   [I asked her] to talk to it about what happened, and [to ask] whether it was [her] fault. This image at least [talked to] her.   She was an unwed mother, she had a lot of stress in her life, a lot of circumstances that really didn't make it the best situation to have a child.   The image in her own mind . . . told her: it was doing well, it didn't hold her responsible; it understood what was going on in her life; and it thought that it was better that it didn't come into life at that time. Now you can say that she's just coming to terms within her own mind, she's rationalizing, whatever, or you can say that she really talked to the spirit of the infant. We don't know what she did.

The result of it was, she didn't feel guilty. She felt better about it . . . I [have] worked with a lot of people [and] I found that people do this spontaneously, but we don't tell each other about it. Whether you identify yourself as a spiritualist or whatever, when I start telling people about this, they say, "Oh yeah, my husband died nine years ago and I talk to him everyday, and get good advice." I found that out from my grandmother, and I found out that this is a natural part of the grieving process.

When people have arrested grieving processes, and they come in very often sick, I encourage them to continue their communication with their image of that person that they're missing. They still have an opportunity to continue to work out loose ends, which they haven't done, and to express their feelings. It's a very powerful, very healing experience.

ONSLOW WILSON: Dr. Harman has been resting his voice. The physicians have been doing all of the talking for the past fifteen minutes or so. We have to get these Ph.D.'s talking [so here's a question], "Dr. Harman, do you access specific states when you fire-walk? Can you access this state at any time to heal, or cure, or to accomplish 'impossibilities'?"

WILLIS HARMAN: To deal with the last part first, yes. All that I can do is tell you anecdotally of my experience of fire-walking, because there's another lesson in there, and it wasn't the one I expected to learn. After two or three hours of preparation, we went out and stood around the fire, about thirty of us, and I was about number twenty-nine to volunteer.

The reason was that I didn't feel in another state. I thought [that I ought to be in an] altered state of consciousness, and I ought to know that it feels different, but I didn't feel anything like that at all. The main thing I was aware of feeling was cold fear. But when I stepped out on the coals, there was really no sensation of burning, or even of heat particularly.

The conclusion that I am forced to (and I don't ask you to believe) is that I didn't really have very much faith myself and I was accurately reporting that to myself, but I walked on the faith of twenty-nine other people, and I think that's a phenomenon, too. It felt to me like a significant lesson.

ONSLOW WILSON: Of course the conventional wisdom would say that it was all in your imagination. Here is a general question to the panel: "What causes six different cosmonauts to see several huge 'angels' out in space?"

WILLIS HARMAN: Maybe because they are there. That's called the principle of parsimony in science. You take the simplest possible hypothesis and go with it.

ONSLOW WILSON: That's interesting, because basically all we're doing really is trying to find some reasonable explanation for our observation. That's basically what it is. If we see six angels there, there is no one ever going to convince us that they weren't there. Now why they were there is a different story. Here's another question from the audience: "Will the physical symptoms, headache, backache, disorientation, etc., ever go away, or at least diminish in frequency or severity, once you have gotten, or are going through therapy, and are working on getting 'stuffed emotions' out and working with them?"

ALAN BRAUER: They certainly can. We certainly hope that they will, and it depends upon the kind of therapy and the person who is getting that therapy. I'm convinced that there are some people who, even though the therapist may know why they have pain, are never going to give it up. [This is so] because pain is their identity, or at least it serves a valuable, what we call 'secondary gain,' and the benefits of having it outweigh the advantages of giving it up.

When we see that kind of situation, there's no kind of therapy that anyone is going to do from the outside that's going to make the slightest bit of difference. On the other hand, if a person is motivated to truly give it up, then it's likely that they will, or at least they can.

ONSLOW WILSON: Good point. Because many times people ask to be cured when really what they're asking for is some attention.

ALAN BRAUER: One way, when attention seems to be the issue, is to assign attention to that person. I'm seeing a lady in her mid-seventies, who is driving her general practitioner crazy because she calls him three, four, five times a week with some concern of pain or some other related complaint. And he threw up his hands and said to me, "Dr. Brauer, you've got to help me!" So I began seeing this lady, and it was apparent that what was happening was that she was in a relationship with her husband, who was giving her attention every time she had a complaint. Whenever "she" called the doctor, more often than not, it was her husband who called the doctor.

There was a dyadic system happening there. Rather than wait for her to have a problem that then forced a very loving and attention-giving husband to do this . . . I assigned her to give a report of her physical condition six times a day to him, at specific times during the day, for five minutes [each time]. Now that was about half the time that she actually spent complaining on her own, or talking to him on her own, but it was assigned. She really resisted that. And I also assigned the husband to ask her [how she felt] at six different times during the day—they were retired and spent a lot of time together—and they resisted doing this, but you know it was an astounding phenomenon.

Within two weeks of this forced exercise, she was having significantly fewer spontaneous complaints, and her calls to her general practitioner had definitely gone down. This has persisted now for [as long as] I've been seeing them—for about three months. So attention can be a really critical phenomenon.

ONSLOW WILSON: This is a somewhat late question but I think it's important to ask. "How effective is a learning or self-enrichment tape on a person when sleeping?"

ALAN BRAUER: It sounds very attractive. Hypnogogic learning—a brave new world! It's been tried. There have been several studies done on this kind of theta wave, possibly delta stage learning. The problem is that it doesn't seem to work. There's a very limited amount of information that can be passed on.

When lists are given, such as names of rivers in the fifty states, there's some evidence that a person may learn to associate some more names than they knew before they went to sleep. But it requires constant repetition. It is very clear that it is not at all an efficient way to learn even though there may be a very minimal amount of information that can be passed along.

WILLIS HARMAN: Can I just add something briefly? That seems to be a perfect example of doing the wrong experiment and coming out with the conclusion that may not really fit. If you use this approach to remove a barrier to learning, then there may be times when it really seems to work pretty well. As far as I know, that's the kind of indication that I get. I am not at all surprised that if you use this to learn fifty rivers when you don't have any motivation at all to learn fifty rivers, then it doesn't work very well.

ONSLOW WILSON: Also, it seems to me that the interaction between the "conscious" aspects of mind and the "subconscious" aspects of mind is a very important factor. Many people are trying to learn, and to get rich by learning, while sleeping. It seems to me that it's kind of a lazy person's approach. That's my personal bias.

ALAN BRAUER: Onslow, you sound like some of my medical school professors who say that in order to learn something you have to really sweat a lot.

ONSLOW WILSON: As I said, that's my personal bias, but here is another question from the audience: "What efforts are being taken to blend the professional counselor, psychologist, allopath, chiropractor, and body-worker into a service community?"

ALAN BRAUER: I was planning on mentioning some of that this afternoon in my talk. Briefly, it can be done—it's very exciting. There are relatively few centers where this is happening. We are trying to do this in our center in Palo Alto, and are finding some really exciting things. It meets with a lot of resistance, of course, from many different sources—both traditional M.D.s as well as even supposedly open-minded lay people. But I think that it really holds one of the keys to the future of healing.

MARTIN ROSSMAN: It's not an easy thing to do, as people say, but it's certainly possible. Ken, with the Psychosomatic Medicine Center long ago in Berkeley, and Behavioral Medicine Unit; Alan's center in Palo Alto; our center in Mill Valley, Collaborative Medicine Center—there has been a lot of people working hard trying to evolve the framework for doing this.

It is very exciting. There's a lot of difficulty [with] people speaking different languages, you know. You get the nutritionist, and the biofeedback person, and the marriage-and-family counselor, and the acupuncturist, and the doctor, and [it] can be a Tower of Babel. But you get the right people, who have gone across disciplinary lines, and are open thinkers, and are oriented in the same way, and there is a tremendous enrichment of learning. And the people who use the services can be beneficiaries of that. Ken has had a long experience in that.

KENNETH PELLETIER: Let me make one observation [which] is that we tried this almost ten years ago, as you know. And I think the clinical model, and the clinical skills have been there. . . . You've done it in your practice [Dr. Rossman], I know Alan has. But to me one of the greatest sources of optimism is something I have learned from working with the business community which is, at this point in time, things that seemed like simply a good idea a few years ago are now being driven by economic imperatives.

I think you can either look at it rather cynically, or look at it as a source of great optimism. I choose to see it as a source of great optimism. And given these economic restructurings and incentives in the medical care system, it necessitates group practices. It necessitates people working together to provide more high-quality and more efficient care. Both of those I think are what is possible, and both are possible in cooperative models.

Let me give you one example. Corporations, in the private corporate sector in the United States, control somewhere between forty and forty-three percent of the total medical expenditures on an annual basis. That means that this year the monies, if you will, in the hands of private corporations run somewhere over two hundred billion dollars. Now they have been very passive and they, by and large, have been forced to select only what Blue Cross, or Metropolitan, or [other] major insurance carriers told them they could have. That's changing extraordinarily rapidly. And as that changes, they develop their own program, and say, "We would rather, with these enormous sums of money, select this program and that program." What they are selecting—and this is by track record with

Xerox and Johnson & Johnson, AT&T—what they are beginning to select are group practices, integrated models that combine physical therapists, psychologists, clinical social workers, [and] physicians into a well integrated system capable of delivering quality care at a reasonable price.

If you will, the economic underpinnings and driving force are now in favor of what simply used to be a nice but not terribly serious idea. And that's only about two years old. Probably the single greatest impact on medical care is the diagnosis related group, or the DRG laws . . . And I don't think we still have figured out, or realized, what the impact of this is on the future pattern, [on] a future kind of provision of care.

ONSLOW WILSON: We are almost out of time, but there are two very interesting questions that I would like to have us deal with before we close this session. The first one is: "Do any of you have any metaphysiological theories in regard to widespread epidemics such as AIDS?"

ALAN BRAUER: I think that we are seeing something that happens periodically in the course of civilizations and the course of time, and that is the existence of plagues and cycles of illness. And so, from the long view of medical history, it's not that remarkable that we should now be experiencing some particular, so-called crisis. Looking on the bright side of what is really a very dismal prospect for what's going to happen in the next few years in my view, with the problem of AIDS . . . is that I think this is forcing us to put attention on what Ken was talking about [in] the area of psychoimmunology, because this is one of the newest frontiers.

It's really been only in the last couple of years that this has been a fit area for research. And there's no question that AIDS is going to push us rapidly into knowledge to understand more about the interaction of the mind and the immune system. I am fundamentally optimistic that we are going to find a way of handling that, but we are going to have some problems for the next few years, in my view.

MARTIN ROSSMAN: I just want to add that [insofar as] epidemics [are concerned], major advances in understanding (at least in culture and often in medicine) usually come during epidemics and wars. It's like the disease model I was talking about when people re-evaluate their lives when they have cancer or heart attacks. We are all looking at maybe we can do that better; maybe we don't have to get to that [crisis] point. We're certainly running out of time; we can't afford to do it anymore with war. We are up against that one, and the same thing may be happening in terms of illness.

Cultures and subcultures will go through those experiences too. Certainly if you have any one of these diseases, and you're identifying with your body, and with that individual lifetime (as most of us at least partially are), this is a tragic and difficult and frightening kind of experience. If you can step back and look at the march of history, and human knowledge, and evolution of spirit, and so on and so forth, my faith is that something very good will come out of it, ultimately, in terms of knowledge.

I think we will probably learn more about neuroimmunology, perhaps from this crisis, than we have in the last [few years or] ever—and hopefully soon.

ONSLOW WILSON: Well, gentlemen, we have run out of time. We will, unfortunately, not be able to deal with that second question during this session; nevertheless I want to thank you for your participation. Thank you all very much.

Chapter Five

PERSONALITY AND DISEASE

by

Brendan O'Regan

Editor's note: Brendan O'Regan, researcher, author, lecturer, and consultant, is Vice President in Charge of Research and also Director of the Inner Mechanisms of the Healing Response Program at the Institute of Noetic Sciences. A neurochemist by training, Mr. O'Regan has, among his many accomplishments, served as Research Coordinator for Dr. R. Buckminster Fuller; as Science Policy Consultant at Stanford Research Institute; as consultant to BBC Television on the relationship between science and religion; and as Associate Producer for the NBC Television Special entitled "Psychic Phenomena: Exploring the Unknown". Among his writings are: "Changing the Images of Man" and "The Emergence of Paraphysics" in Psychic Exploration, *edited by the astronaut and founder of the Institute of Noetic Sciences, Edgar Mitchell.*

Mr. O'Regan, who addressed the April 18, 1987 Symposium at Pasadena City College, is therefore no stranger to the changing paradigms in science which constitute a veritable New Heresy.

BRENDAN O'REGAN: Thank you. I hope you can hear me. Well, it's a fascinating time to be talking about these subjects because so much, as Willis [Harman] pointed out, is indeed changing. I think back to the fact that in 1975 when I first began working with the Institute, one of the first jobs I had to take on was administering a grant to Carl and Stephanie Simonton to look at the work they were doing with terminal cancer patients. They were using imagery, such as Marty Rossman has just described to you, with patients.

People came to us not infrequently and said, "You guys must be totally crazy to think that the mind has anything to do with a disease like cancer." The climate of opinion at that time was deeply opposed to such linkage. It certainly made no sense to people that these linkages existed, or that the mind could in any way affect the course of an illness, but we knew that effects were happening to patients.

I believe that if you're going to be scientific, in a real sense, the first thing you have to be is phenomenologically open. You've got to be willing to say, "Is there an effect, even if I don't understand it?" and if it's there, [you have to] begin to at least examine it and deal with it. That's what we try to do. Of course, at that time there was a lot of information lying around that had not been coordinated and put in one place. One of the areas that was there as a clue to all of this for anyone who was open enough to look at it, was the whole area of what is commonly known as the placebo effect. The placebo effect, as I'm sure you all know, is what happens when a patient is given something that they are told is a drug or a powerful means or method of healing but which in fact is an inert substance—sugar pill, saline water, or what have you.

They proceed to respond as though a powerful drug has indeed been given to them. To give you some sense of this, I'd like to read a short piece to you which is a description of one of the more famous cases in placebo that actually was written in 1957 and published by Dr. Bruno Klopfer. He's talking about a patient named Mr.

Wright who had a generalized far-advanced malignancy involving the lymph nodes and lymphosarcoma:

> He developed resistance to all known palliative treatments as well as severe anemia, ruling out the use of x-ray or nitrogen mustard. Huge tumor masses the size of oranges were in the neck, groin, chest and abdomen. The spleen and liver were enormous. The thoracic duct was obstructed and between one and two liters of milky fluid had to be drawn from his chest every other day.

> He was taking oxygen by mask frequently and our impression was that he was in the terminal state, untreatable other than to give sedatives to ease him on his way. In spite of all this, Mr. Wright was not without hope, even though his doctors most certainly were. The reason for this was that the new drug he had hoped to come along and save the day had been reported in the newspaper. Its name was Krebiozen, subsequently shown to be useless as an anticancer agent.

> Wright had hoped to be included in a trial with Krebiozen, but his physician refused as the drug supply was limited and to be used for patients with at least a few months of life remaining. Wright pleaded for the drug, his enthusiasm boundless, and out of pity his physician agreed to include him in the thrice weekly injection protocol.

> Mr. Wright, febrile, gasping for air, completely bedridden, received his first injection on Friday. By Monday, Mr. Wright was found to be walking around, chatting with patients and staff. His tumor masses were halved in size—a more dramatic regression than the most radio-sensitive tumor could display under heavy x-ray every day. It could only be described as brilliant progress. Within ten days of his first

Krebiozen injection, he was discharged from the hospital.

Two months later, news reports on the effectiveness of Krebiozen began to appear; it was ineffectual. Coincident with these reports, Mr. Wright relapsed and was readmitted to the hospital in his original state.

Seeing an opportunity to double check the drug using Wright as a control patient and knowing of nothing else that could help, the physician told Mr. Wright that he would receive "a new super refined double strength product." Anticipation was built by delaying a few days ostensibly waiting for the new shipment to arrive. With much fanfare, the injection of sterile water was finally injected.

Recovery was even more dramatic than in the first instance. Becoming the picture of health, he again remained asymptomatic for two months until the final AMA [American Medical Association] announcement that Krebiozen was a worthless drug for the treatment of cancer. Mr. Wright was readmitted to the hospital in extremis, his faith gone now, his last hope vanished, and he succumbed in less than two days.

So, you might say that placebo effects are not something to ignore—they can be dramatic. Of course, the other thing that happens with placebos that people don't often pay attention to is that they can have side effects. And that's something that we don't try to think about or explain.

There's a fascinating paper in the World Journal of Surgery in 1983 which was a routine report about a new chemotherapy. As you know, the standard thing you do is you have a control group that you give a placebo to because you think they don't do anything—we know better—and you have an experimental group to whom you give the drug.

Now in the content of this paper there's no mention made of what I'm going to tell you other than in the table describing the effects. You have one table describing the effects on the patients of the drug and another column describing the effects on the patients of the placebo. And what is very curious is, if you study the paper, you'll see that thirty percent of the patients getting the placebo lost all their hair.

Now, you begin to wonder. There is a sense in people's minds; they know that chemotherapy is supposed to make you lose your hair. One can only wonder what sort of mechanism might have been operating that the expectancy of these people thinking they were receiving chemotherapy was so intense that they obliged by losing their hair. You could say that they're having all the side effects of chemotherapy and none of the benefits, which is really unfair.

Another story in this regard was told to me by Bernie Siegel at Yale, who was talking to me about the change in effectiveness of drugs over time. There was a specific one that he mentioned, called cis-platinum, which was once regarded as a very promising treatment for cancer. And when it was first being administered, they were getting something like a seventy percent effectiveness rate using it. But, by the time that the treatment began to be administered by people not as enthusiastic and as excited and close to the source—they were saying, "Well, here's the latest thing for you," and they gave chemotherapy in a rather routine fashion—the effectiveness rate dropped to something like thirty percent.

So there seem to be very powerful mechanisms operating here that can tune the system and can allow it to function very differently. We began to get interested in that and wondered how much that was really a factor in healing in general. Of course, another way that we began to be aware of this plasticity of mind and body—I think it was

Marty [Rossman] who talked about the plasticity of the system; this whole relationship between mind and body is a very dynamic thing that can move in dramatic ways—we began to look at people with multiple personalities.

Now, you know a little bit about this, I'm sure. All multiples are people who have a major dominant personality and then whole hosts of sub-personalities that split off. The reason that people are multiples is a tragic one: all multiples are people who have been severely abused, physically and sexually, over a number of years. Not all people who are abused become multiples, but as far as we know, all multiples are people who have been abused.

What they are doing, in effect, is they are dissociating in their minds to escape from the reality that they have to live with. Why we got interested, in a very particular sense, is that multiples display a whole range of phenomena that could teach us a great deal.

For example, multiples are known to be allergic to a drug in one personality and not allergic to it in another personality. They are known, for example, to not only have different drug reactions but different susceptibilities. They will seem to be, for instance, alcoholic in one personality—I know of a case at Rush Presbyterian Hospital in Chicago where a patient was diabetic in one personality and not in another and they could literally watch the change happening in insulin levels and so forth as the personality switched.

There are more strange cases of women who have three personalities and three periods every month because each personality is linked to a different cycle. There are cases that are reported that are a little harder to deal with where personalities change and eye color changes—which is kind of curious.

Another major thing that happens, by the way, is that the EEG (the electroencephalogram) of a multiple can change radically between one personality and another. Dr.

Frank Putnam at NIH [National Institutes of Health] has done a major study of this and found that the EEGs of multiples switching from one personality to another are as different from one another as if you had taken the electrodes off one person and put them on another person.

What is very interesting about this is that, you know, the biology is the same—at least the genetics are the same; it's the same person physically. This change in personality is going on and it changes the whole tuning of the whole system, if you like.

We're sponsoring a study at NIH—it's ironic that Noetic Sciences gives money to NIH to do certain things, but that's what you have to do sometimes when you want to persuade people to do things in a different way—we have a program going on there where they are studying what happens to the immune systems of multiples when they change personalities. I believe this is the first time this is ever being looked at. We reckoned that the immune system must be involved and if they're displaying an allergy in one personality and not in another, some immune mechanisms must be changing profoundly, and we're trying to find out what those are.

The whole [point] . . . that is buried in that story is that finally we are beginning to really notice that the brain and the immune system are linked. The history of immunology has always been caricatured as the headless body. The immunologists didn't really work with the study of the immune system in a way that required it to be connected to the nervous system and so they noticed that it seemed to be able to function without that. At least with cellular immunity they could look at what T cells can do in the test tube and they could look at what macrophages do in the test tube and so the link to the brain was the last thing to be noticed.

It is very interesting to me that when I was sitting around with Carl and Stephanie Simonton back in 1976 [I was] saying, "Well, you're getting these effects, what do you think—how do you think it's happening? What system do you think is mediating these responses when you alter the psychological environment of the patient and the spiritual environment of the patient? How do you think it's coming through and manifesting in their physical condition?" They published at that time a model which said that they felt that the likely site of impact was the immune system.

At that time there was no field of psychoneuroimmunology in any formal sense. I think I attended my first meeting on the subject at Stanford in 1981. Today we have a rather different picture going on because it is now known—and Marty [Rossman] talked about some of this—that, for example, widows or widowers experiencing grief following the death of a spouse have depressed immunity for many months.

Stress in college students, who are of course, the paradigm for all major research, does show examination stress, [which] changes IgA and IgG levels and so forth. So, these kinds of linkages are beginning to be looked at, at this point, and are beginning to be mapped.

We thought, however, Let's take a plunge into an even more dramatic body of evidence for all of this. I borrow a quote here from Norman Cousins to introduce this idea. "Over the years," he said, "medical science has identified the primary systems of the human body: the circulatory system, the digestive system, the endocrine system, the autonomic nervous system, the parasympathetic nervous system and the immune system. But two other systems that are central to the proper functioning of the human being need to be emphasized: the healing system and the belief system. The two work together. The healing system is the way the body mobilizes all its resources to combat disease; the belief system is often the activator of the healing system."

So we have operated from the premise in our Inner Mechanisms program that there is in fact an unknown, undiscovered healing system that lies dormant until stimulated into action by stress, trauma or disease; and it comes in, does its work and then leaves; and we sort of bump into it when we have a placebo effect.

I thought, Well, the placebo effect is a generalized demonstration of self-repair capacity, self-healing ability, in the human being. Then I thought, What body of evidence is there that is a more dramatic demonstration of that? We decided to start looking into the medical data on spontaneous remission that Willis [Harman] mentioned. Spontaneous remission has had a rather checkered history in medical science. The majority view is that it is an artifact of misdiagnosis; you didn't get the diagnosis right the first time, the person never really had that illness, and of course, they now seem not to have it because they never had it in the first place. Now that, to me, is dodging the facts.

The first serious study of spontaneous remission was published in 1966 by Everson and Cole in which they looked at 176 cases of regression from cancer. They distilled those down from a thousand reports that they [had] obtained. Then you have no further major publication in the literature on this topic until, in 1974, there was a conference at John Hopkins University on spontaneous regression of cancer which was published as an NCI [National Cancer Institute] monograph in 1976, and since then you have no formal publications, no texts, nothing. It is not talked about in medical school and it is very difficult to do research, as we found out.

For the past year and a half at the Institute we have been conducting a major survey of the medical literature on this topic. And it has taken us a year and a half to now assemble, in hard copy, three thousand reports on spontaneous remission, from over eight hundred different medical journals in twenty different languages for all kinds of disease.

We now have volume one of a document that will be published later this year. All kinds of cancer and all kinds of cardiovascular diseases, allergic disorders, gastrointestinal, pulmonary, hepatic, endocrine, you name it, it's in here. I won't say that everything has been known to remit, but you'd be surprised how many diseases are listed here. When I show this to physicians, it tends to stop the conversation for a while because people just have not had the opportunity to see this put in one place. And, of course, the first line of argument is, "Well, where did you get these reports?—Oh, the New England Journal of Medicine." "Oh, Cancer." "Oh, the Journal of the American Medical Association." I mean it's actually all in there, in establishment medical journals. We're not telling them anything that hasn't been published in medical journals; it's actually all there. What it's saying, however, is that some rather amazing forms of self-repair can go on. And it's essentially invisible; we don't really know why. Now, when you start looking at this literature, some patterns do begin to emerge which are very interesting.

First of all I have to say that, because of the climate, doctors have to be pretty courageous people to write a paper on remission because they first of all have to go into meticulous detail about the diagnosis and the reconfirmation and they must do the x-rays again and the slides have to be reexamined and the histology repeated and it goes on and on. Each of these papers is sort of written as though no one had ever tried to do this before and it becomes this litany that you get used to as you start reading these papers over time. Then they have to do the same thing all over again about the disappearance because it just simply is not expected.

Unfortunately, because of that focus, you rarely get much about the patient, much about the person to whom this is happening, and of course, that's one of the things that you deeply want to know about. You do get little clues, however, which are sort of interesting. There's one paper that I remember by Dr. Weinstock in New York whom I spoke to a few weeks ago about this subject. This was a woman who had cervical cancer that had metastasized throughout her body and she was really expected to die in a few months, two or three months, and he continues on in the paper and says, "And her much-hated husband suddenly died whereupon she completely recovered." You know there must be some connection; wouldn't you think? But there is no study of that, you see. This is the problem.

We then went to the National Cancer Institute [which] operates something called the National Tumor Registry. They have eleven centers around the country and if a person goes to a hospital and is diagnosed with a particular type of tumor, the Tumor Registry in that area is informed because that is how the epidemiology of cancer is basically tracked.

We went to the Bay Area version of this, the Bay Area Tumor Registry, and said we were interested in spontaneous remission and they said, "No, no, we don't know anything about that." I sort of took a deep breath and said, "Well, how about long term survivors?" And they said, "Oh, yes, well we do track those." And I said "Okay, a survivor for you is someone who has survived free of cancer for five years." They said, "Right." I said, "Well, how about, let's look at not five year, but ten year, survival."

"Let's go into your data base." This conversation took place in 1985; their data base was computerized in 1973, so I thought, Well, let's deal with the computerized record. I said, "Let's look at the number of cases you had diagnosed as terminal with metastatic illness between 1973 and 1975, and see in 1985 how many of those people are still alive." That's ten years and it is metastatic illness and it's a terminal diagnosis; it's a rather stringent set of criteria.

In fact the question was, Would there be anybody? And the answer was that there were a hundred people.

They were quite taken aback by this. They were not expecting to find this little nugget in their own data base and I wasn't either, but, you know, something said there should be something there. And one of the things here is that there are all sorts of nefarious things that go on with whether or not people have really died, and whether people are still trying to claim insurance, and Medicare, and all kinds of stuff. So there's a bit of fraud here in the death statistics that you have to overcome.

That meant that we had to fund them [the Bay Area Tumor Registry] to go back in and verify that these people were in fact alive. They found that a couple had in fact died and a few were lost to follow-up, so we ended up with a residue of eighty-nine people.

What's very interesting, what astonished me, was that two of these cases were severe pancreatic cancer, which is a rapid killer. It normally kills people very quickly and yet here were these two cases of people still alive ten years later. We are now in the process of going through the necessary protocols to get permission to identify these patients (with their permission and so on) and to interview them, to start talking to them, to find out what they would have to say.

Of course, we have interviewed a few people in remission because now we're beginning to hear about this. People are coming forward to us saying, "I know somebody." A lot of people have come up and said, "I'm in remission, I'm okay." And we are proceeding now to prepare to interview these people on videotape.

I remember the first couple of reports that we had from these people. A woman had cancer and her first question to the interviewer (who was Caryle Hirshberg, the lady at our Institute who was doing the primary gathering of the data) was, "You're not a doctor, are you?" And Caryle said, "No, will that be a problem?" She said, "No, I don't want to talk to doctors, they've told me I was wrong so many times that there's no point in my talking to them."

There is a little message in this. Many people in remission are lost to follow-up in the medical system because we don't receive their information very hospitably. That's something to know more about or to search for and we're going to have to be careful how we do this; we don't want to rock the boat with these people, we want to inquire in a gentle way and say, "Tell us your story, what did you do?"

There's a funny anecdotal story here: A woman we know who is doing research on this advertised in the paper in Moscow, Idaho—was there anybody out there in remission? She got twenty-five replies and one woman was a farmer's wife and she came in and then Glenda Hawley, who's doing the study, asked, "Well, how did you feel when the doctor told you you had terminal cancer?" Her answer was, "That was **his** opinion." So, [we see] this attitude of independence. Hawley said, "Well, how do you mean?" She said, "Oh, we have these experts that come and tell us things all the time; government fellows come to the farm and tell us that our crops won't grow unless we do this and that, but hell, we just put the seeds down and things grow anyway and nature takes its course." So there is this picture emerging of a kind of autonomy and independence in these people, and I think that we have to begin to respect that.

We have many cases, for instance, in the data base dealing with remission that occurs concurrently with intensive meditation. There's a whole series of papers from Ainsle Mears in Australia on the regression of cancer in association with intensive meditation and we will be publishing many of those references.

Another area that I've looked into is the area of miraculous healing because I thought to myself, Well, where is there a lot of extraordinary data on this? We were looking through the journals and it was scattered pretty thinly.   I thought to myself, Lourdes is a place where people have claimed miraculous healing for a long time. Since 1858 there have been six thousand claims of miraculous healing in Lourdes, of which only sixty-four have made it through to be miracles.

Here you get into an interesting distinction. The medical commission at Lourdes' first line of questioning on a claim of healing is, Could it be a remission?   And if so, they throw it out because they consider that to be a natural—not a supernatural—phenomenon.

Little did I realize that when we publish this, [which is] the largest study ever done on remission, we will affect the criteria for the evaluation of miracles at Lourdes because we know of things remitting that they didn't know about.   Their charts are going to have to be changed because [of] several things that they think are miraculous; they didn't know of reports of it remitting with people who didn't ever go near Lourdes, or had no involvement with the Virgin Mary or what have you.

Another thing: I said, "Well, you know this apparition appeared in 1858, is there anywhere that this could be going on now in the world?"   And the answer is yes.   In Medjugorje, Yugoslavia, there is a little village where some several million people have been.   It's not talked about in this country, [but] an apparition of the Virgin Mary appears every day.

I went there about a year ago to see what this was all about.   The thing is that I was considered an anomaly there because no one had come there to find out about healing.   Was miraculous healing going on?   People were coming there for pilgrimage reasons, for very sincere reasons of devotion.   And, one of the things the apparition is saying (which doesn't make people very happy in the hierarchy of the Church) . . . is, "People should become aware of God in their own way."   And those [last] four words do not suit the doctrines of the Catholic Church, but they do happen to be what the apparition is saying to the children.

There have been some 250 to 300 cases of extraordinary healing there. By the way, when you walk around there and see that many people in intense devotional states, you cannot but notice that there must be a hormonal reflection and an immune system reflection of what this is like.

Since the immune system is a terribly abstract thing for many people, I want to show you quickly some images. . . . I have slides of that and I also have some images from patients' drawings, paintings of their illness and so on and I want to kind of bring these two kinds of images together so you can see.

I want to first show you some of the basic pieces of the immune system and then show you what some of it actually looks like because it will, I think, trigger some questions in your mind that will make you realize that the immune system is a sensory system itself. We tend to think that we have the five senses and some people argue about six and seven of the psychic or other kind. But when you look at some of these images, you will say to yourself, How is that seemingly blind cell knowing that there is something very far away from it over there, and reaching out and grabbing hold of it? It's a very interesting thing to just make that a little more concrete.

You'll see here [on the slides] just a mention of the various elements. The macrophages . . . engulf and digest debris in the bloodstream. Encountering a foreign organism, they communicate to the T helper cells and get them to come to the site. The T helper cells . . . identify the enemy, rush to the spleen and lymph nodes where they stimulate the production of other cells to fight the infection.

Killer T cells . . . activated by the T helper cells, specialize in killing cells of the body that have been invaded by foreign organisms as well as cells that have turned cancerous. The [B] cells . . . reside in the spleen or the lymph nodes where they are induced to replicate by T helper cells and then to produce potent chemical weapons called antibodies. The antibodies then move from that site to the site of infection.

Then there are suppressor T cells, the third type of T cells, and [also] memory cells, and I won't get into the details here on those.

What do we have here? At the top you see the cancer cell and these little white fellows are killer T cells advancing on that cancer cell to attack it. Then you'll see that when they get closer they change shape, (they elongate) and they attach and they start doing their work. So this is a real science fiction battle going on inside you.

When the cancer cell is dead, this is the fibrous cytoskeleton that is all that is left of the cancer cell with a presumably happy little killer T cell just sitting there saying, "We got him." Here's a closeup on that T cell and you can see it's just surrounded by the debris of the dead cancer cell.

Here is not a killer cell, but a T helper cell. The blue specks that you see all around it are the AIDS viruses attacking that cell. It's interesting to realize the difference in scale and size between these two. These little dots—each dot—is an AIDS virus, and that's the size of the [much smaller] AIDS virus relative to the size of the T helper cell. What's interesting, just so that you understand the implications of this, [is that] there's some very important work that's happening at NIMH [National Institute of Mental Health] at the moment where Dr. Candace Pert has identified the exact site, the exact receptor site, which is just a tiny little area on the surface of the T cell where the AIDS virus attaches to attack it and take it over.

That's quite a feat of modern science because—look at the size of the virus—they know exactly what piece of the protein coat of the virus attaches to the exact piece of the T cell. Curiously enough, the same site is the site attacked by the Epstein-Barr virus which is becoming very common and chronic Epstein-Barr infection is something to reckon with these days.

Interestingly enough, they've also designed a peptide, an eight amino acid long peptide, that sits in that site on the T cell and blocks the virus which is potentially a very important treatment for AIDS . . . The U.S. government has patented it as long ago as last August, [but] has yet to do even one clinical trial of it in this country, although it has been tried on four patients in Sweden, one of whom is in complete remission, and two others are seemingly okay.

We wonder about this supposed rush program of the government to test these things. . . . They're really not doing anything, at least, not at the speed that they could be. What's interesting here is that these peptides are also the mediators of emotion and here's the link that Marty Rossman was talking about: the T cells have receptors on them for all the neuropeptides that are found in the brain, so the brain and the immune system are very tightly linked.

On an evolutionary basis, you wouldn't expect receptors to be on the T cell that wanders around if it weren't needed in some way to communicate with the brain. So one wonders if in fact the stimulation of emotions is not stimulation for the production of neuropeptides that in turn act on cells of the immune system to instruct them in one way or another. I think this picture is going to emerge in much more detail.

Here is one of the other examples I wanted you to see. This is a macrophage: the big white thing at the top, and this is a bacteria down at the bottom. You'll see that it's reaching out to grab hold of this thing and get rid of it

and it obviously has a mechanism of sensing it. This is
what's called a pseudopod which is coming out to engulf it.

These macrophages are pretty active fellows and they
will not just go after bacteria. Here is a macrophage
extending out and these are little droplets of oil. [The
macrophage] is sending out pseudopods to grab all those
too because they recognize it's "not self." It's foreign
debris so they will go after it. They will even, in fact,
commit suicide. There is a macrophage attempting to
absorb asbestos fibers and it will die in the process but it
automatically recognizes that that shouldn't be there and it
attempts to clean it up. Here is a macrophage extending
pseudopods to E. coli bacteria to get hold of them. This is
the initial phase of the process; and then later they have
engulfed them—they are inside—they're being all sort of
sucked inside of the macrophage. So this is all very
dramatic stuff that's going on inside there, unknown to us.

This is a B cell dividing. And then we talk about self-
repair; here is an example. Those red cells are red blood
cells and the white is fibrin that is building over it to heal
a wound and there is actual self-organization of that whole
system going on without our involvement.

This one is not so relevant to this lecture, I guess. It's
malaria protozoa replicating and the membrane breaking
open releasing the parasites. So you get an idea that it is,
I think, interesting to see what is going on in there.
When we're talking about these things in the abstract,
sometimes you need to know what they are doing and that
they have a life and an intelligence, of sorts, of their own.

Here are some children at M. D. Anderson Hospital
playing what is called the Killer T cell Game. These are
cancer patients who are using a computerized version of
this to stimulate their imagination of the T cells killing
cancer cells.

I happen to think this may be a mistake because it is
externalizing as a technology what should be going on

internally as imagery from inside. As Willis [Harman] points out we get a certain kind of science [and] we tend to do a certain kind of thing with information. I'm not so sure it's the right thing in this case.

I reemphasize this statement from Norman Cousins because we're talking about the role of the mind in both the conscious level and the unconscious level. Our belief systems are certainly not all conscious. They are partially conscious indeed and whole portions of them are unconscious.

You know, even if people are given the intellectual or social pressure to change a belief, it's difficult for them to do so sometimes. It doesn't matter whether you are talking about prejudices against different races or different religions and so on. Even when people know intellectually they ought to not feel that, they have trouble changing it because there are unconscious components in there. So I thought it would be interesting to look at some images from patients about what they believed about doctors because that should determine something about what they think doctors are going to do to them.

These are some images: here, "The doctor is depicted as a heartless sadist who scourges his patient, a small pathetic figure." Some of these are extreme, but they do convey something of how people feel in the medical setting. A patient feels like a freak at a fair. "See the nude woman; nothing's sacred." . . . "Students come along and say, 'Oh, can I look at this?'" and the dignity of the person is challenged.

Here is a painting by a patient: "I would like a good doctor I can trust." And you see it's a lonely figure seeking help and so forth. "The Cliff of Depressions" was another painting by a patient with depression and [it shows] how difficult it was to overcome.

These next slides are from Bernie Siegel's recent work. When asked to draw her doctor giving her therapy, [the patient] drew the devil giving her poison. She also portrays her disease as an insect, a negative image considering how hard it is getting rid of insects. In fact, when patients come up with insects as the image for their cancer, it is not a good sign. Here's a closeup of that image, and you can see all kinds of things are built into that, I mean, there's the cancer, there's the notion of the devil and there's the skull and crossbones and all the imagery is there.

"This woman was honest enough to show her conscious despair at the need for chemotherapy, indicated by the sad face and black outline. However, there is a symbolic message for her from her unconscious telling her to receive the treatment; that it is good for her. The syringe is purple, a spiritual color, and her feet are turned toward the therapy. The image convinced her to try the treatment and it was successful. Her fears melted away with the tumor."

These next slides, from *Art and Healing,* by Edward Adamson, are images that patients have of themselves: "help me," supplication, prayer, guilt. People in the hospital feel that they somehow should be guilty for being ill; they need reassuring that their illness is not a punishment. This was a self-portrait by an artist who had severe depression, and it's a complicated image of a crying plant weeping onto itself and so forth. . . .

These are how people see themselves. "The whole person represented has all the assets to make herself change. She has good self-esteem indicated by the size of the figure on the page. She stands in a neutral position, hands at her side, with her hands ready to get a grip on things. I'm concerned about the ever-present smile, however. How do we respond when someone asks, 'How are you?' or 'What's going on in your life?' Symbolically, the smile is a performance, like answering, 'fine,' or 'nothing.'" If we perform, we wear ourselves out for the sake of others. Being happy is fine, but performing is self-destructive.

This is just another way in which we're not often allowing people to express [themselves] and so they tend to repress.

This is an image this woman drew of herself being boxed in, another idea that when people are in the hospital and removed from familiar affection from family or spouse or what have you, they need more of that [affection]. They need it replaced in some way.

"This is someone who is sitting down on the job, only giving half of herself; her disease again is depicted as an insect, a negative symbol. Treatment is black, bringing despair. It is not entering her body, showing non-acceptance."

I wonder, if you would ask that person what they thought, whether they would have given you as much information as this image seems to contain.

Here is an interesting one: this man talks a great deal about healing through love. His white blood cells are carrying his cancer cells away; he couldn't even bear to kill them. So he's just taking them out and he's going to drop them off somewhere. There's an interesting thing that Siegel says here: "I feel that images of attacking the disease may work for about twenty percent of the patients, but eighty percent need a different approach to heal."

I don't know what Marty [Rossman] will say about this in discussion, but I've been encountering a number of points of view [in] which people are now saying it is more important for the patients to be asked to come up with their own imagery, not to tell them to imagine it as white knights or this sort of thing. And, of course, Marty's story was exactly that: the patient came up with the image of the fist that turned into the hand and so forth. That is a refinement in our thinking about imagery these days and that's why I partly wonder about this TV-computer game with these children. I don't know if that's feeding into the right circuitry here to get good results to happen.

This [slide] is a closeup of the working leucocytes; it says, "Boy, I'm sure glad these duds are leaving. It will take us weeks to clean up this mess."

These are more complex images and I don't think I'll take the time now to go into these, but you can get a lot of the patients depicting their situation, how they feel about their disease and the world in general. . . . Some of those are from *Love, Medicine and Miracles* [by Bernie Siegel] and others are from another book called *Art and Healing*. I can give you references later if you want.

So you know, when you sort of get inside this whole process and you see the life in the immune system and what's going on in there, we begin to wonder. It's a very complicated situation and it's not that simple, but at the same time, it is not surprising that all these linkages are being found.

What I want to do in the remaining time is just say that we may be at a very important juncture because I think that we may be about to reconceptualize how a lot of diseases occur. I'm thinking here of the work of Candace Pert. If it turns out that really the receptor sites on the T cells are one of the major places where an attack occurs on the system and produces the distortions of immunity that then allow cancers to develop and so on, if we're now beginning to map all those sites and if we're beginning to find out what kinds of peptides (nontoxic substances) can go in there and help the patients, we may be on the verge of really reconceptualizing exactly how this whole thing works.

Candace [Pert] has already manufactured a series of these peptides and it looks, for example, like schizophrenia may be reconceptualized as the immune system attacking the nervous system because of wrong instructions or possibly a viral induced condition. Certain kinds of cancer may yield to this kind of thinking. And it's very interesting when we try and put these two things together. I want to give you a quote from Ernest Rossi who has written a very good book. . . . I strongly recommend his book, *The Psychobiology of Mind/Body Healing,* because it tends to pull all this together in a very intricate way. He says, for instance:

> Thus the slower acting, more pervasive, flexible, and unconscious functioning of the neuropeptide activity of mind/body communication more adequately fits the facts of hypnotic experience than the faster acting, highly specific, consciously generated processes of the central and peripheral nervous systems. If we were to use a computer analogy, we could say that the peripheral nerves of the central nervous system are hardwired in a preset fixed pattern of stimulus and response just as is the hardware of the computer. The neuropeptide system, however, is like the software of the computer that contains the flexible, easily changed patterns of information. The receptors and highly individualized responses of the neuropeptide system are easily changed as a function of life experience, memory and learning. Neuropeptides, then, are a previously unrecognized form of information transduction between mind and body and may be the basis of many hypnotherapeutic, psychosocial, and placebo responses. From a broader perspective, the neuropeptide system may also be the psychobiological basis of the folk, shamanistic, and spiritual forms of healing that share many of the characteristics of hypnotic healing currently returning to vogue under the banner of holistic medicine.

So, what one is finding here is a way to kind of make sense of these effects. And we don't have to throw the effect out because we don't have the mechanism. In fact, really, the effects are challenging us to have more sensitive methods of looking for mechanisms of connection between spirit, mind and body.

I do feel, however, that—and I am taking note of Willis' [Harman] four-tiered model of science—we shouldn't fall into a new reductionism by thinking that that's the whole story. And I think that it's when you start reading some of the case reports of the miracles at Lourdes that you begin to realize that there may be another order present on some occasions.

A fascinating story is that of a man named Vittorio Micheli who was a miracle cure at Lourdes in 1976. We're talking about something rather recent and so the potential for misdiagnosis is less and the potential for advanced treatment is greater and so on. He had a sarcoma of the pelvis and it literally was eating away the pelvic bone. The hip had dislocated from the pelvis and the patient was in a full body cast, could not walk, [and] had been in the hospital for something like a year. He was taken to Lourdes at his request and immersed in the water, as all the patients are. Some people say that the real miracle of Lourdes is that no one has ever gotten sick from drinking the water in which all these bodies are immersed every day. . . . He felt something that you will find throughout many cases of extraordinary or miraculous healing, an electrical sort of charge, a sensation of, well, the best word we have for it is like an electrical charge. I suspect it's probably something slightly different than that, but I don't know. He had been nauseous, he had been unable to eat, he had all kinds of gangrene problems setting in and he was really in a very advanced condition. I have, by the way, the complete medical report on him, including the x-rays before and after and I have them here if you want to look at them.

He was immersed in the water and immediately felt better, I mean, immediately. He felt this current go through his body and he immediately felt better. The doctors, however, at Lourdes are a little blasé because they see so many people who do not get healed; it is still rare to get healed there. "60 Minutes," if you saw that ridiculous program they did on Lourdes, will tell you that they managed to do a whole program on Lourdes and they didn't interview one person who was healed! And there are thirteen of them alive and living in France and Spain and Italy, you know. So much for investigative journalism, I think.

Anyway, this man was taken back to the hospital and they finally re-x-rayed him one month after he was at Lourdes and were amazed to find that the bone was reconstructing and they realized that something really had happened. Two months after being immersed in the water, he was up and walking, with a slight limp, which he treasures as his memory of the fact that he did have a severe illness at one time.

Another one that I'm looking into at the moment which is very intriguing, is of a woman in Pennsylvania who had multiple sclerosis for twenty-five years and had her last medical examination confirming that condition in May of 1986. She heard of Medjugorje, the site in Yugoslavia where the apparitions are appearing. And she read a book about Medjugorje (written by René Laurentin, a French Jesuit who is one of the Church's major scholars on miraculous phenomena) called "Is the Virgin Mary Appearing in Medjugorje?" It's sort of an investigative report on the whole thing. In that book, of course, it talks about what the apparition is telling the children who see her—six children see the apparition, rather similar to how Fatima and Lourdes occurred. And the Virgin, of course, is saying that she's appearing because the world is in great danger and that there will be major catastrophes and that people should return to an awareness of God and so forth. But in the book, he says the message of Medjugorje's [is] that people should return to an awareness of God and pray and fast. And the fast is not a very rigorous fast even.

So she decided to do that. And she was doing that for a month and didn't notice anything in particular and then she reread the book and realized that she'd forgotten to ask for healing for herself. She'd really been asking to do God's will; she had not been asking for anything for herself. (Kind of an interesting story [is] there that I could expand on if we had time.)

That night she included in her prayer a request for healing. She felt something (an electrical charge again), that thing that seems to happen, but didn't notice any major change in her condition. She was taking a class at a college and she had a special car [so] she could go there and she was wearing braces up to her hips and these crutches, short ones. She was sitting in this class and she suddenly began to realize that her left toe was itching. She had lost sensation in her feet eleven years before. By the end of class she was completely focused on the fact that she could wiggle her toes and she thought, My God, something is happening.

She went out to the car and realized that her legs didn't look right because her knees were no longer bent in, they were straightened; she took the crutches off and was walking. [She] ran to her doctor—actually she ran to her priest first, to tell him—and then to the doctor who burst into tears and said he had never seen anything like this. We're investigating that case at the moment.

So, you say to yourself, "Hmmm, there's remission of the kind you work for and you do the kind of deep inner work that you have to do and there seems to be something else that happens on occasion. It may be rare, but it does occur." So I think that we should recall all of this and realize that we are making major advances but there's still more to learn.

And I would like to finish by reading you a poem from Rilke, Rainer Maria Rilke, and it's interesting to know something about Rilke. This is from the "Sonnets to Orpheus" and dedicated to the memory of a young woman whose premature death deeply affected him. "These strange sonnets" Rilke wrote, "appeared, often many in one day, completely unexpectedly. I could do nothing but surrender purely and obediently to the dictation of this inner impulse." And one of those sonnets [XIX] is:

Though the world keeps changing its form
as fast as a cloud, still
what is accomplished falls home
to the Primeval.

Over the change and the passing,
larger and freer,
soars your eternal song,
god with the lyre.

Never has grief been possessed,
never has love been learned,
and what removes us in death

is not revealed.
Only the song through the land
hallows and heals.

Thank you.

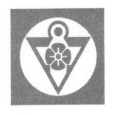

Chapter Six

STRESS AND THE SUBCONSCIOUS MIND
by

Alan Brauer, M.D.

KRISTIE KNUTSON: I am now very pleased to reintroduce, once again, someone who is a friend of ours by now. Dr. Alan Brauer is a diplomate of the American Board of Psychiatry and Neurology. He is currently the Director of The Brauer Medical Center in Palo Alto, which specializes in treatment of stress and pain. Dr. Brauer is the founder and first Director of Stanford University's Biofeedback and Stress-Reduction Clinic, and is a Clinical Assistant Professor at Stanford University in the Department of Psychiatry and Behavioral Sciences. Dr. Brauer is also an active member of the medical staff at Stanford Medical Center, and is a well-known expert in the field of stress control, and is a pioneer in use of biofeedback. He has participated in over 250 television and radio programs across the United States, Canada, Europe, and Japan. He writes and lectures extensively on stress management, aging, sexual therapy, and expanding human potentialities. Will you please join me now in welcoming Dr. Alan Brauer.

ALAN BRAUER: Thank you. Can you feel the energy in this room? This is a great experience. Most groups don't have this kind of energy. Just feel it for a moment, just take it in.

Most of the time when I'm talking to professional groups, there is a sense of skepticism and hostility. But in this situation it seems to be a little different; it's the dropping of limits. And I really want to thank Dr. Wilson for being able to put together this kind of a group of people, both the presenters and the audience, because there is a real sense of possibilities. Your questions are great. And with this kind of sense about what is possible, the kinds of breakthroughs that Ray and Marilyn are talking about will happen sooner [see Chapter Eight]. Where do these breakthroughs come from? Well, they don't come from deliberateness; that's a really important point. If you set out to discover something, you won't find it. So where does discovering creativity come from? Well, it comes from some place that we can't name, like the unconscious. So one of the things that I want to talk about today has to do with the unconscious, which is really the major part of our mind.

Most of the time we live in the conscious; at least that's where we think we live. But all that happens to us, happens for the most part . . . from unconsciousness. So we've got to know something about that. The other part of what I'm going to be talking about is related to stress.

Stress is a really important topic these days. It's very pop. Everything now is related to stress, stress diseases "I'm under stress." "Sorry I'm late. It's because I'm stressed." "I can't go to work. I'm stressed." "My marriage isn't working because I'm stressed." "I can't talk to my kids because there's too much stress." We throw this around very easily, but really we don't have much sense about what it means. And with good reason, because, frankly, nobody really knows exactly what it means. It's a really loose term, although it started out as being precisely defined. Actually, it started out coming from the field of engineering.

Hans Selye is the inventor in the field of stress, and he conceived the effects that pressure can have on systems. But because Selye was Canadian, it's thought that he used the wrong word. He used the word stress, but really he meant strain. So really the whole field of stress and stress-management should be strain and strain-management. But we're stuck with a bad translation. Stress, in the engineering sense, is the force that's applied to an object, and that's a precisely measurable force in pounds per square inch, for instance. Strain is the effect that force has on a system. That can be measured also. So Selye conceived that he might be able to quantify the effects of pressure on living systems. He made some important discoveries. His discoveries, though, were made on animals subjected to very precise kinds of stress—not exactly the kinds of things that human beings are likely to experience. What did he do? He put animals in centrifuges, gave them low doses of poison as the stressors, and still he found some quite interesting things. Primarily, he discovered that organisms respond in very predictable fashion to the effects of these kinds of stresses; that almost regardless of the kind of stress that was applied, organisms had a set series of reactions—actually, three kinds of reactions.

The first is the fight-flight, and this is when the organism gets all geared up to deal with an emergency. That's an absolutely normal kind of reaction, and is essential, and it happens to us hundreds of times a day, and it's nothing to be concerned about. On the contrary, it helps us to survive.

But what happens if this stress continues? Then the second phase sets in, which is called, according to Selye's paradigm, the stage of resistance. In this, the body continues to deal with the stress being applied to it, but it digs in; it's set for a longer seige. It's not just a car cutting in front of you on the freeway, and you go "damn," and then you go driving along. It's when the pressure remains, and it remains, day in and day out. The body starts secreting hormones, and muscle tension increases to try to deal with the pressure being put on it. Oftentimes a person is not even aware that this second phase is occurring because they get used to it.

Now our systems are only human, and after a while the third phase sets in, which is the phase of "uh-oh, exhaustion." Do you know about that phase? This is much more serious because systems actually begin to break down. Here you find failures of the various organs in the body, such as ulcers that may begin to bleed, hearts that begin to fail and cause heart attacks, clotting mechanisms that become overly active . . . and cause strokes that can result in death. This is called the general adaptation syndrome, and [is] something we all need to understand because we are all subjected to it. Our bodies were not designed to spend time in the second and third phases. That is, we are not supposed to experience this phase of resistance or exhaustion. If you are there, you've gone too far. But the problem is that we can't help it, or at least we think we can't help it. And the way our lives exist, for virtually all of us, forces us to deal with being exposed to not only the first, but the second and the more serious third phase of stress because we can't get away from the stressor.

Our body-systems are brilliantly designed to deal with this first emergency phase. That's why our blood pressure goes up; that's why our muscles get really tense to get ready to run away or, theoretically, club an aggressor. But you know what happens if you try to club a cop who stops you; you may feel like it, but you might only get one shot at best. Then you'll be paying a very heavy price of stress for a long time afterwards. So we're forced to deal, in a chronic way, with forces that our bodies are not designed to take. So we have to figure out how to cope with this unnatural process. Fortunately, we do have a mechanism, and we have to look to our minds and our consciousness to find a way out. We'll talk about some of the ways in which we can use our consciousness and unconsciousness to un-stress our bodies and get ourselves healthier.

Well, how is it that there seems to be a problem? How is it that we don't automatically deal with stress better? Well, that's a complicated question, and it has something to do with the belief-systems that have developed over many, many hundreds of years.

We have heard a lot today about the problems of getting through our negative beliefs, and how science resists change and discovery at the same time that it is invested in changes and discovery. It's kind of one of those paradoxes. As soon as a new idea is put out, science mobilizes to attack it and shoot it down. This is certainly true in the field of medicine. I agree doctors may be the last to be agents of change in the new consciousness. I'm always having to be aware of the medical model, and the medical establishment, which is heavily invested in a concept called the dualistic theory, which we heard mentioned several times today. This is a pervasive belief that is really stifling change. It's based on the idea that we have a body, brilliant with many extremely complex chemicals and interactions. But this brilliant body has a mind that is disconnected from it. We have a brilliant mind as well, but there is no relationship between the two. This is the dualistic theory.

Now who invented this dualistic theory? It was none other than René Descartes, who certainly was brilliant in his investigations at the time. But what's ironic is that this philosopher should still be influencing our thinking four hundred years later. Do you realize how rapidly knowledge is changing? It's doubling every twenty years. Well, how can we be allowing ourselves to be influenced by a concept that one time may have been useful, but isn't now; all the evidence is pointing against it. Everywhere we look, we're seeing all of the exceptions to this split between mind and body. We all kind of scratch our heads and say, "Well, yes, but that's an exception." Many others who have talked before me have pointed to these kinds of funny things that exist, that should make us scratch our heads and wonder. And we do, but then where do we go? You see, until you have a new system to move to, a new belief system, you cannot abandon the old. You'll continually plug up a leaky boat until you have a new one. So we've got to find a new system that helps us understand how our organisms operate.

We're getting close when we're looking, as Ken Pelletier was pointing out, to the mind/body connection. There is a lot of exciting work happening in how we are connecting our thinking and our bodies, how that is being bridged. I believe that the more we look at this bridging process, the more we are likely to come upon a third type of experience that is different from mind, and is different from body, and is different even from the bridge between the two, a third kind of consciousness that there's really no name for at this point. Carol McMahon, who is an M.D. doing some work in this area, calls it the Biotonic Concept. [That is] probably as good as anything else, although it still remains to be elucidated.

This has something to do with the idea that basically we are an automatically self-regulating system; that if we just let our systems be, we will experience our highest potential. If we try not to monkey with the mechanism, our mechanism will work perfectly. But it's this monkeying process that keeps getting us into trouble. It's our thinking that messes us up. It's the way in which we are living that causes us to do things that are really destructive to us. If we could somehow allow our natural regulating process to take over, and live in the most natural kind of state, then we would experience the highest level of health possible and the highest level of consciousness. So we need to figure out how to get to this natural state.

In order to get there though (since we're in an interim phase, we're definitely not at that level of consciousness yet), we do have to still do some monkeying with the mechanism. So we do need to use our conscious minds to help give us some clues, but we are not to rely on that consciousness. So it may well be a dentist who helps make this breakthrough. Actually, creative discoveries have been shown scientifically to occur at random times, but not entirely random.

There was a study done about fifteen years ago of the activity most associated with creative discoveries. This was before the women's movement, because it was shaving, and I believe that it was facial shaving. So there's something about having the mind in a relatively neutral, automatic place that allows the creative process to happen. And indeed, one of the important essentials of getting our bodies into the most healthful place is to be able to turn off that overly busy conscious mind, and also the unconscious mind, which is where there's so much damage caused, but also where lies the greatest hope.

What is this unconscious mind? The unconscious mind consists of the automatic regulating functions of the body. So this part of our mind controls heart rate, blood pressure, muscle tension, breathing, hormones, all those kinds of automatic functions that we take for granted, but which, incidentally, can become controlled if we want. The other essential part of the unconscious is related to memory. Do you know that every single experience that you ever had in your life since you were born, and perhaps before you were born, is recorded in your mind? It's like having a permanent video tape running all of the time. So we have these hundreds of billions of bits of data that are stored in here. And that means that we can access, potentially, anything that has ever happened to us.

We have to know how to access it because [the unconscious mind] just doesn't necessarily produce the data we want at the moment that we want, but it's available if we use our conscious mind to help guide us. Of course, what also follows from this is that much of what comes up from this permanent memory storage are data and memories that may not necessarily be in our best interest; they may not be related to our best health, or our best way of relating to the world, because they include all kinds of negative messages, all kinds of bad experiences, painful experiences.

Every time we are exposed to something painful, that's recorded. So if a bully smashes us in the face when we are four years old, we may develop a fear of other people because other people may, in fact, have been at one time dangerous. We also record all of the negative messages that we hear from people that are important to us, such as parents, teachers, and friends: "You must be careful, watch out, the world is dangerous." "You are a failure." "You are going to be sick just like your dad." "You'll never make it in life." "What you need is to find a good husband and settle down. You don't need to go to school." All of these kinds of messages get in there and are recorded, and unless we know what's there, we are likely to be influenced by those. So we have to have some way of knowing which of these experiences are coming up to our subconscious level and influencing us.

I want to share a little bit with you about how I got to be interested in some of these things, because these are not usually the areas where good, conservative physicians put their attention. We should be passing out pills and worrying about DRGs (Diagnostic Related Groups). I was a busy intern at Bellevue Hospital some fifteen years ago, and I was alarmed to discover that I was developing a blind spot in my right eye. This was fairly alarming to me so I consulted an ophthalmologist, who said, "Oh yes, you have central serous retinopathy." That sounded both good and bad; at least there was a label to it, and that's always a good thing. The bad thing, though, was that although in theory there was a treatment for it which sounded hopeful, it was a laser treatment—and that's really nice of modern technology coming to the rescue—but the problem was that the particular location of this leakage in the vessel that causes a retinal detachment was in an area near the central part of the eye that couldn't be operated on with this new laser technology. "But what causes this problem?" I asked him (and, subsequently, a number of other ophthalmologists) because I didn't like what he said. He said, "Oh, it's stress. So you have to get less stressed." Well, here I am in the middle of an astonishingly tough internship where I am on call every other night and average about three hours sleep a night, have no time to think, let alone figure out how I'm going to get less stress. What am I going to do, quit my internship? Go off to Fiji? But this was the ophthalmological consensus. So I worried about that some.

The eye got worse until I saw an announcement for something called Transcendental Meditation. It sounded kind of fluky and hokey, but it sounded awfully good at the same time, so I went to hear this lecture. It sounded really neat that you could use your mind to control all kinds of astonishing things in your body, so I became a meditator. And, amazingly, within just a few weeks after practicing this technique, the deterioration in my eye stopped. That really felt excellent. Plus, meditation felt really good. I wasn't sure I was doing it exactly correctly, that's one of the problems; it just seemed too simple. Of course, they throw in all of these other parts of the process, you know, the oil and the other trappings. I suppose that's helpful because it helps give weight and credence to the process. Being a good scientist and also being kind of lazy, I stopped meditating after this good development happened. Within a number of weeks the leakage and the blind spot resumed. So there was further evidence, and then I became hooked. I was just meditating away like crazy—I'd go to the bathroom and I would meditate in the hospital aisles.

Several years after that I found out about an interesting kind of process called biofeedback. And this sounded wonderful also because here was an electronic way of accomplishing the same thing. Now one of my favorite things as a kid was playing with electric trains. I had a basic interest in electronics, and here was a way to take the technological developments and apply them to this kind of fluky-seeming meditation process. So I bought a biofeedback machine, began using it myself and started to think that there must be a lot of ways of using this new process. At the time I was a first year resident at Stanford, and although Stanford has accomplished many things in research, at this point it definitely had accomplished nothing in the field of consciousness-change or biofeedback.

I had to sneak in the first biofeedback instrument to use on my first patient, who was an engineer who had headaches and depression. I thought that maybe if I could use the instrument on his headaches that would be an important, useful thing. Indeed, his headaches pretty well stopped after about four or five sessions, and much to my surprise, also, his depression lifted even though I was spending much more time on the biofeedback than I was on the good therapeutic strategies that should have been employed at helping his depression. Somehow this process of learning how to control his physical system not only eliminated his headaches, but made him feel better. It may have been a sense of success; it may have been that he was depressed partly because of the headaches; it may have been because he was handling his stress better and, therefore, less depressed because he was defusing the stress rather than absorbing it. And so I became really a proponent of this use of machinery to help bridge our minds and our bodies.

Biofeedback is indeed a brilliant model for this bridge between our minds and bodies. It was not the panacea that the first biofeedbackers put out, because you cannot just get yourself hooked up to a machine and get biofeedbacked to health. It takes something more than that; it really takes a context in which this happens. It takes knowing how to use the process that occurs. So you can't just go out to Radio Shack and buy a little GSR. If so, we'd all be perfectly healthy. Right? Because you could get biofeedback machines at Radio Shack for $14.95.

A third interesting thing happened to me, which we already mentioned today, and that was the experience of fire-walking. How many of you here have done that? Just almost none of you. Boy, you have an experience in store for you. Just step right outside, we have a fire going. No kidding. . . . It really is an astonishing thing. Of course, we have all read about fire-walkers, and it just sounds like something literally out of this world, and I had always thought that you needed to be a professional fire-walker to do this. When the opportunity presented itself at one point, I went to simply observe this fire-walker do his thing, and found myself in the position of being kind of "under the gun" to consider doing it myself.

It was definitely not the intent that I had in going to this; I was just going to be a scientific observer. But it's really interesting when you're faced with something that you know intuitively that you should, or could, be able to do because there's no question that the fire-walker was able to do it. There was also no question that a lot of people who tried doing it had gotten burned. And as a matter of fact, one person who had gotten burned was a man that I know that specializes in consciousness and its exploration, a man you all know and have probably read his books. Since I knew for a fact that he had gotten cooked, I was understandably a little hesitant.

At the same time I knew that I was committed as an adventurer, and researcher, and practitioner of pushing limits; I was going to need to do it. There was, of course, the question of making sure that you are in a sufficiently deep state of altered consciousness as Willis Harman pointed out this morning. How can you be sure? I didn't have my biofeedback machine with me. I think there was some help that there was a full moon out, because it gave something to focus on above. Essentially the process is—somebody, I think, this morning asked the question about how do you do it—the process is to visualize yourself accomplishing it. It's very important, in this and in anything you want to accomplish, to picture how you want it to be as if it's now, and to picture the process of accomplishing it, step by step. Also, it is important to get into an altered state of consciousness because it is in the subconscious state that we can rely on our bodies to be at their optimum. See, we have to trust our bodies to know what is best.

Walter Cannon wrote about the wisdom of the body. We have to trust our bodies, however they know, to be in the optimum state and to take care of us. Because this process, if you're going to deliberately test it walking on hot charcoal, is going to require that you really have that kind of belief and faith. Belief is a critical part of getting into the optimum state. You have to have correct belief, which is a positive belief, or at least an accurate belief.

Then, of course, there are a few other little tricks in fire-walking, like—keep walking! Also, when you're finished walking, wipe your feet because there may be little cinders under the feet. And so, trying to keep these several things in mind, I then took the plunge, walked across, and it was really less of a push than walking on a beach on a hot day; it was really amazing, it's easy. Anyone can do it! Well, literally anybody probably can do it if you just go through those steps. It's not as difficult, or as frightening, as it may sound.

This was an important event in my experience because it confirmed what I really knew and believed. But every once in a while you have to have an experience that confirms what you know to be true because, otherwise, you kind of lose faith, you forget. And that's why it's important to give yourself pep talks a lot, also to talk to other people who have gotten through these blocks and impasses, and to come to workshops and seminars like this, to look ahead to the future, and also to reaffirm what you already know.

For quite a while after this fire-walking had occurred I found myself even better able to communicate positiveness and belief to patients that I was seeing, because that's really a critical part of helping people get better.

Right now we're talking about stress and what that is. These days it's considered that virtually all illness is stress-related. The reason this concept has become so popular is because of the problems that medicine has had in dealing with illness. Most G.P.s [general practitioners] and generalists who see the whole spectrum of diseases know that the vast majority of patients that they see really have nothing wrong with them. They may have symptoms but they are not symptoms that medicine can treat. The main way that medicine treats is with medication and with surgery. Most illnesses that we have cannot be treated with medication or surgery.

Yet all of us want help and so doctors are stuck. We're expected to do something and yet there isn't much that we're allowed or can do. So we try the best that we can. If a patient wants medication (which most people seem to want, although somewhat less so these days) and we don't give it, then we make them angry. They are just going to see another doctor, or they are going to think that we are a bad doctor, or their anger is going to make the symptoms worse.

So at least give them something that is not going to hurt, and that will help. But the problem is that it really doesn't help, and can often make the problem worse because many stress-related problems, in fact, are made worse by medications because they cause problems of dependence if you are giving any kind of tranquilizers. If a person has constipation and you give medication for constipation, you may make the problem worse because you are going to get a rebound effect, and yet, something needs to be done. Doctors are kind of stuck. After a person who has a problem goes to more than one—often five, ten, fifteen—doctors to get some help, they finally realize that they may not get real help from the traditional medical profession. They may feel that their problem needs to be handled by a different method so they go to alternative healers, acupuncturists, chiropractors, nutritionists and homeopaths.

In fact, any or all of these so-called alternative methods can be equally effective. Because what we're looking at, for most symptoms and problems, is not a purely physical problem, and it's not purely an emotional problem. It doesn't all exist in one's mind or in one's head. And we do need to do something. The concept of a stress disease then becomes very helpful because here is a way of labeling a problem, giving a diagnosis and a potential solution.

Stress-related illnesses really are almost all the illnesses that we get. Of course the common ones that we associate with stress are ulcers and asthma, and high blood pressure, and psoriasis, and hives, and things like that. But essentially any kind of a symptom that we get is going to be aggravated by stress; it has to be because stress is, by definition, too much pressure on our systems that pushes our systems out of whack, and therefore, makes lower our ability to fend off illness.

AIDS is a worse problem than it might otherwise be because of lowered immunity. There is good evidence that people who have high levels of immunity are less likely to contract AIDS, even when they have the virus in them or have been exposed. We know that a related kind of problem, which is the herpes virus, very definitely is affected by the mind. So it becomes important to have our minds operating at their optimum level so that our bodies can be functioning at the optimum level as well.

There is so much more I want to tell you. . . . I really want to suggest that each one of you—since you all have been exposed to these ideas of the value of emphasizing the unconscious and of the bridge between the mind and body—do some kind of mind/body bridging, some type of self-regulation process. The simplest way of doing this is with any one of the many kinds of relaxation methods, or imagery methods. But do something absolutely regularly every day, and when you find yourself with a problem, use this skill that you have, or will develop, to focus on that problem. Trust your subconscious to come up with the best way of handling that problem and you'll find your minds and your overall health getting better and better. Thank you.

Chapter Seven

HEALING AND THE SUBCONSCIOUS MIND
by

Onslow H. Wilson, Ph.D.

KRISTIE KNUTSON: Ladies and gentlemen, here once again is our dear friend Dr. Onslow Wilson. For those of you who were not with us first thing this morning, I just want to once again share with you that Dr. Wilson is the Director of the Department of Instruction with the Rosicrucian Order. He is a biochemist and has done specialized work in immunochemistry; and he is the author of the book *Glands - The Mirror of Self*. Will you please join me now in welcoming Dr. Onslow Wilson.

ONSLOW WILSON: You know when I was growing up, my parents told me that the sign of a good host is to put himself last. And I've always adhered to that but I must confess that there are certain disadvantages, because you get the remnants. And so now here I am; I really don't know exactly what I am going to say to you. I have a few slides that I may or may not use, but maybe I'll brag a little about the Rosicrucian Order.

All of the things that you've been hearing here today are things that the Rosicrucian Order, for centuries, has been teaching its members to do for themselves. Who is the physician anyway? Is it Dr. Brauer, or Dr. Rossman, or Dr. Whoever who gives you the placebo? Or gives you the confidence that you can cure yourself? Or is it an aspect of yourself? That's really the essential question, I think. For the Rosicrucian, when it comes to matters of health, the thing we are concerned about is addressing the physician within ourselves. That does not mean that if we don't know exactly what to do, that we should not consult a conventional physician; that's not what we're saying. But we are saying, that in the final analysis, healing comes through the internal, or interior, physician. So why spend a lot a money and why go through a middle man? Some of us need to. It's a kind of ritual that we have built into our own minds, so we need to. So please don't think that you're going to leave here, and throw all of your old habits aside because you have attended a Rosicrucian sponsored symposium on Metaphysiology, because that's not the way it works.

The Rosicrucian Order knows that it takes time and we, in the United States in particular, we have instant breakfast! When we have a headache, we go for "instantine"; when we turn the television on, bang! the picture's there; when we turn the radio on, bang! the music is there, rock-and-roll or otherwise. So we have grown accustomed to expecting instantaneous results. When we do not get instantaneous results, we become just as instantaneously frustrated. We limp from one frustration to another, going from one physician to another, when the real physician is as close as our very skins. That close—closer than your very skin! That's where the real physician is. So one of the things that the Rosicrucian Order does is assist its members in learning how to address that physician, or that other aspect of ourselves which, from the scientific point of view, is at least three and one-half billion years old, compared to thirty-five or twenty-six or seventy-six years old.

There are a couple of things I would like to share with you in terms of our own researches, and these are things that come primarily out of our research laboratory which is headed by Dr. George Buletza who is in our audience today. For any of you who are interested in further information about what I'm going to tell you, you may address him directly. I claim no responsibility for this except perhaps a little twist as far as interpretation goes.

One of the things we are concerned about is a healthy body. Why? Because we can only realize our fullest potentials in a healthy body. The idea was thrown out today that disease, or illness, may be the Western way of meditating, or learning a little more about ourselves. It's an interesting idea. But it's almost as though we are saying that we have to be ill in order to learn. I am not sure that is necessarily the case. But anyway, we do fall ill from time to time because, consciously or otherwise, we have introduced disharmony between what we may call the two phases of mind, which is the outer and the inner. When this disharmony manifests, it soon manifests in the physical body because, from everything we have been hearing today, there is a very intimate connection between the mind and the body.

Now we've heard about imagery. Dr. Rossman talked about imagery, and the imagery he described was imagery generated within the mind of the subject him or herself. I want to talk a little bit about the influence of imagery held in the mind of others on behalf of the subject who is suffering, the subject who is ill. We have not touched upon this at all. We have made allusions to it by saying that support groups can make a difference, and I think in one of the latest newsletters of the Institute of Noetic Sciences there is an article on healing the mind/body/spirit connection, I think written by Brendan O'Regan. And in there, an article is cited regarding the influence of prayer on behalf of people who are ill. I think there were 393 people who had heart problems, and these patients were randomized by computer, using the computer process, and so nobody knew who was going to be receiving prayer and who wasn't; it was a double-blind study. It turned out the people who received prayer, the people for whom prayer was indulged in, suffered less, far less complications. I don't recall the exact statistics but those of you who are interested can find this in the newsletter of the Institute of Noetic Sciences.

We, over the years, have accumulated a dossier of innumerable testimonials from our members who have either received spectacular assistance in the sense that they suffered less; or required no medication, or little medication compared to others; or even the most dramatic of all instances—spontaneous remissions. This assistance is rendered by a group here at Rosicrucian Park, which convenes every day at a given time, and simply visualizes things like thoughts of peace, love, harmony, kindliness, health, and so on. That's all! We do not have to visualize white cells gobbling up cancer cells, for example. It's a very general visualization. What we're doing is assisting the person or persons who have requested this assistance; we are assisting them in experiencing a sense of wholeness.

Because when you think, and live, or visualize, or temporarily place your consciousness totally in harmony, peace, love, you are experiencing wholeness; there are no divisions; there's no disharmony. When you do that, you can experience healing, depending upon how sincerely you really want to be healed. Because as we said this morning, there are people who ask for assistance, who pray to God, who do "all the visualizing in the world," and still don't get better. Is it enough simply to see a picture in your mind? Is that enough? From our point of view, the answer is no. You must live this picture, you must become emotionally involved with this picture. If you are not emotionally involved, nothing is going to happen. You have simply sat in front of a television screen and walked away. You have to be in the picture.

So, when our members request assistance, because there are times we do need the assistance of others—as the saying goes "No man is an island" but that was before women's lib, so now we can say, "No person is an island"; I think it's perfectly safe to say it that way—so we do need the assistance of others from time to time. What happens is that the person requesting assistance is expected to cooperate with us. They have to be receptive to what we're doing. If they are not receptive to what we're doing, then nothing happens. So the fact that we have this tremendous dossier of testimonials is indicative of the cooperation of the member, not so much anything that we do as a group, but the cooperation of the member in turning his or her consciousness over to the internal physician.

Now this all sounds very speculative, and sure they wrote a letter saying, "The doctor said, 'Boy, did you heal fast!'" This is a very subjective piece of evidence. Science demands proof. Why? Because with proof comes confidence. When you have confidence, then nothing is impossible. That is really the essence of science, at least for me. So I want to show you a few slides. I want to show you two in particular, dealing with the influence of imagery held in the mind of others on behalf of a subject who has requested assistance. The reason I need to show this is because we want to give you the confidence that these things do work. And when we see graphic proof, then we say, "Yeah, well this is not just belief anymore; it is really true."

In the body there are electrical polarities. I don't know how many of you are aware that the body has profound electrical polarities. The work of Burr and others prove this beyond doubt. As a matter of fact, the polarities in the body are such that the center of the body is positive relative to the periphery. The right hand, generally speaking, is positive relative to the left. The back is positive (we were talking about electrical polarities now), the back is positive relative to the front. The head is positive relative to the feet.

What we did was, we got a subject, and you see the degree of polarization between right and left is an indication of the degree of stress that a subject is experiencing.

I want to digress a little bit and say something about stress. I think that there is a general misconception about stress. Stress, or chronic stress I should say, is really a situation that evolves out of a sense of low worth, low self esteem. We don't have the confidence that we can deal with a situation. Imagine, for example, you have a job and your boss is a son-of-a-you-know-what, but you need the job because if you quit, you don't know where (at least that is what you'll tell yourself) you don't know where you are going to find another job, and your kids have to be fed, you have got to have milk on the table—never mind bacon, but milk—and here you are, and this boss is you-know-what.

What are you going to do? . . . You cannot fight your boss, and you cannot run away. You are stuck! And, because stress comes out of the so-called fight or flight reaction, you are stressed. Stress, this type of stress, this chronic stress, comes out of the sense of feeling stuck. And when you feel stuck, what you're saying to yourself is you can't do anything about it. And underneath that, you're saying you do not have the confidence, and you don't have the wherewithal to do anything about it. So stress says a great deal about our belief systems, hidden belief systems that we hold deep within ourselves, about ourselves.

So the business of body polarity is indicative of the degree of stress that a subject is undergoing at a given time. And I think the numbers fall out to indicate that between three and five, seven millivolts—Dr. Buletza can correct me if I'm wrong—that this is a normal situation. Anything above ten millivolts is considered to be indicative of a stressful situation. So we had this subject who came in, and was under a great deal of stress as measured by this body polarity, because he indicated, I think it was about fifteen millivolts, between thirteen and fifteen millivolts of potential difference between the right and the left hand.

We simply asked him (I should say Dr. Buletza and his staff simply asked), this subject to sit and remain in a relaxed, receptive frame of mind. At the same time an arrangement was made with the group that does this visualization for assisting people, to visualize a person (the person was not identified) and send these thoughts of peace, love, harmony, etc., to this person. A computerized recording system recorded what happened.

You will see that this individual came in with a right to left side polarity difference of approximately fifteen millivolts, (Figure 1, page 176) which indicated that he was under a great deal of stress. Now during the control period, which lasted fifteen minutes, you can see that the body polarity didn't change a heck of a lot. But the bar [I] on the top, with the arrow just below the left extremity of it, indicates exactly the time when the group began to visualize peace, love, harmony, etc., on behalf of this particular individual.

You can see that immediately the body polarity, the difference between right and left diminished significantly, and when the group stopped visualizing for him specifically, he went back to his rotten ways.

But look at what happened subsequently, when the group decided to do its general visualization for everyone, not just specifically for this person [bar II]. He responded again momentarily, and then went back to his rotten ways, and remained there until the group finished, when he responded again. So he was not entirely insensitive to what was going on, even though out here, objectively, he did not know what was going on.

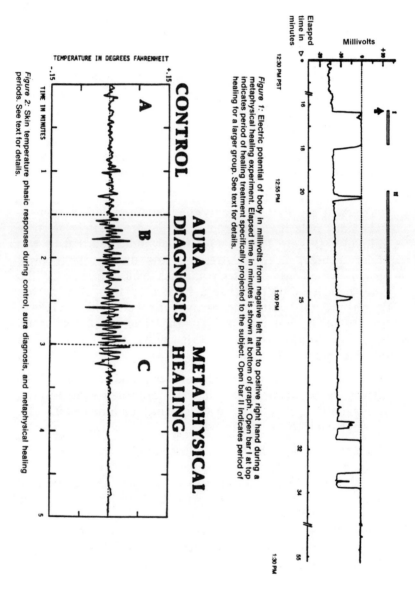

Figure 1: Electric potential of body in millivolts from negative left hand to positive right hand during a metaphysical healing experiment. Elapsed time in minutes is shown at bottom of graph. Open bar I at top indicates period of healing treatment specifically projected to the subject. Open bar II indicates period of healing for a larger group. See text for details.

Figure 2: Skin temperature phasic responses during control, aura diagnosis, and metaphysical healing periods. See text for details.

Notice that he stayed that way for a while, and fussed around a bit, until about thirty-one or thirty-two minutes into the experiment, when suddenly his body polarity goes up into the normal range and stays up there for a little bit, and comes back into the abnormal range and, finally at around thirty-four minutes he goes up, and stays there for the duration of the experiment, which means that he stayed that way for approximately twenty-six minutes, at which point the experiment ended. This we interpret to mean that this person experienced a healing, in the sense of having his stress reduced significantly.

Now why all this bobbling around? We'll get to that in a minute because I have another slide to show you, another experiment to share with you and you will see this kind of bobbling around. We have to interpret that, and I'll give you my own personal interpretation although Dr. Buletza, who actually did this work may not agree with me. But it's my personal interpretation; it makes me feel good.

The next experiment I want to describe to you was also conducted here in our research laboratories by Dr. Buletza and his staff. And this has to do with body temperature. Now we generally think body temperature is so-and-so and it stays rock steady. Well, that's not true, it fluctuates about a mean. And body temperature is controlled by the hypothalamus to which some people refer as the emotional center of the brain.

What Dr. Buletza and his staff did was as follows: they had a member who is a psychiatrist who loves to do what is called metaphysical healing or spiritual healing, and he had his own particular visualization process. His visualization process involved having a rose bush represent the emotional nature, or the emotional state, of the individual that he was trying to help. But before he allows it to represent the emotional state of the individual he's trying to help, he has a preconceived notion as to what the perfect rose bush looks like. So he conjures up in his mind this perfect rose bush, and then he says, "What will this rose bush look like if it represented the emotional state, or nature, of the person I'm trying to help?" And lo and behold, bang! the rose bush would change, and it would develop irregularities at certain points, and these points he had, in his visualization, identified with what some people call chakras (and we could get into a long discussion about the distinction between chakras and what Rosicrucians call psychic centers but we will not. That's not important for us at this point). But he would allow certain positions on this rose bush to represent the location of chakras, that's the term he used.

In his visualization he would just travel up the rose bush and try to harmonize these irregularities. In other words, make them go back towards the ideal state. And while all this is going on, all that the subject is doing is sitting in another room totally unaware of what the psychiatrist is doing, because all that the subject is asked to do is to sit and remain in a receptive frame of mind.

As a matter of fact, I think sometimes the experiment was conducted with no subject at all, just to be sure. You know, one never knows, it may be a quirk of the equipment. It's the scientific method folks, you have got to do it that way. And so this is what this psychiatrist would do, and so I want to show you the result of one such experiment (Figure 2, page 176).

We see that during the control period, labeled "A," there is substantial fluctuation about the mean as far as [the subject's] temperature is concerned. In the section "B," referred to as the diagnostic period, or aura diagnosis (this is when the healer, the psychiatrist, is visualizing this rose bush going back to its perfect state), you will notice what happens. There is tremendous agitation there. And then the psychiatrist stops after he has completed his visualization. Then the next phase ["C"] is what we call metaphysical healing. But you notice the agitation continues for a little while after the psychiatrist stopped his visualization. So here again we have this, what I'm calling "futzing" around. What does it mean?

You will notice that after he's done his thing, his "futzing" around, he settled down and the fluctuations about the mean are very tiny compared to what the subject came in with, so again we see this as a confirmation, or visual proof, that some sort of healing took place because the subjects always reported that they felt so much better, and they really don't know what happened, but they felt so much better, etc.

The "futzing" around as I'm calling it (and I hope no one is offended by this term, sometimes I use such terms and people say, "Oh, he's really getting off on funny words here"), from my perspective what we are looking at in this jumping around and indecision and so on, is a reflection of the decision-making process which takes place at the level of the subconscious. Others have been using the term unconscious, but the decision-making process is taking place there, because all of this is being controlled by the subconscious mind. We do not consciously control body temperature. If we had to be consciously concerned with regulating body temperature, keeping the heart beating, keeping the kidneys filtering, keeping the lungs breathing, and white cells doing what they do, and so on, we would go crazy. We couldn't exist; that would be it.

So the subconscious mind is what is responsible for all of this. And so all this fluctuating about, at least from my perspective, is an indication of the decision-making process that is taking place at the subconscious level. Why must there be a decision-making process? Because the person that lives inside there [the subconscious mind] which doesn't often get to see the light of day out here, has to decide whether or not this is a serious matter. Are we [the subconscious phase of mind] going to change things, then find out two minutes later that this guy [the conscious phase] has changed his mind, and has gone back to his old rotten ways? So from my point of view, this is what is taking place.

So we here, at Rosicrucian Park, have indicated, at least to our satisfaction, that the images held in the mind of others on behalf of subjects requesting assistance have profound influences not only based on the testimonials of our members, but also based on this type of objectively verifiable result. Now while we're in this frame of mind, I have a request from a gentleman in the audience that we send out these thoughts of peace, love and harmony to a young girl (her name is Lynne) for a healing. But what I would request that you do is not necessarily personalize it for little Lynne, but send it out as a general emanation to everyone who needs healing at this time. So if you will, could you invest a few minutes in doing this, please.

[PAUSE FOR GROUP MEDITATION]

Okay, I think that should just about do it. Now when I came to the podium, I wasn't exactly sure as to what I was going to say to you. And when I say "I," you are naturally aware that I am speaking of the "I" that dwells out here most of the time. The other "I" apparently knew fully well what was going on.

The next slide is what I call my "nervous cat" (Figure 3, page 181). This is a representation of the types of responses that take place in the body, physiological responses that take place in the body, when the hypothalamus of the cat is stimulated electrically with electrodes. And you will see a number of very important parameters that have changed with such electrical stimulation. For example, the heart exhilarates, digestion is inhibited, blood is shunted to the muscles because we are getting involved with the fight or flight reaction here; there is a release of sugar from the liver; there's increased oxidation which means that the thyroid gland has been stimulated; there is quicker coagulation of the blood because if you are going to fight or run away, you might get hurt and you don't want to bleed to

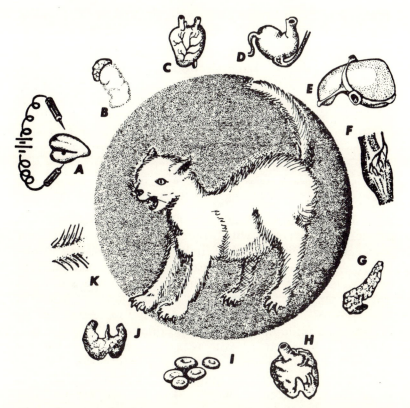

Figure 3 — Direct electrical stimulation of a certain region of the cat's hypothalamus (A) leads to an emotional reaction referred to as "sham rage " In this emotional state there is a generalized discharge from the sympathetic arm of the autonomic nervous system (ANS), resulting in profound effects on many of the body's vital mechanisms. These effects include increased production and release of adrenalin from the adrenal glands (B); increased rate and force of cardiac contractions (C); inhibition of digestion and intestinal motility (D); increased release and utilization of sugar involving the liver (E) and pancreas (G); increased blood flow to muscles (F); increased oxidation involving the lungs (H) and the thyroid (J); increased rate of blood coagulation (I); hair standing on end (K). (See text for further discussion.)

death; and if you have any hair, it will stand on end; adrenalin is secreted and whole hosts of things take place.

This is for the cat whose hypothalamus has been stimulated by electrodes. What electrodes, figuratively speaking, do you use when you get yourself stressed? I think, as Dr. Brauer has pointed out, it's your thoughts; your thinking habits are the electrodes that you use. And "negative thinking" will always produce this type of result. On the other hand, "positive thinking" will produce quite other results. But what is negative thinking? I would like, in the very few minutes left, to leave you with a little thought as far as negative thinking is concerned.

If, in your thinking and your reacting to things, you are concerned primarily with yourself—in other words, your view of things is extremely limited—that is negative thinking. Why? Because you are defining yourself in very narrow limited terms. Any time we become "stressed" in a chronic sense, it is because we are defining ourselves in very limited terms. That, at least in my understanding of Rosicrucian philosophy, is negative thinking. Now you will find, and I put it to you as a challenge to try it for yourself, that if in any situation you seek a solution that will benefit the largest number of persons possible you won't be so stressed. Why? Because you are defining yourself in much larger terms. And what is it we call love anyway? It is concern for others. That's how we manifest love, isn't it? So whenever you find yourself thinking in terms of very limited goals, things that are going to benefit you personally and, perhaps, just your little family or your little group or what have you, from a Rosicrucian point, at least in my understanding, that is negative thinking.

When you can think of solutions that will benefit the largest number of persons possible, that's positive thinking. Those are the stimuli, those are the electrodes that you use to stimulate your hypothalamus. The hypothalamus controls the activities of the pituitary gland, the pituitary gland controls the activities of a host of other glands, but most importantly, the hypothalamus is very much involved in this business of stress, with the release of what is called ACTH, adrenocorticotropic hormone; this hormone stimulates the adrenal cortex to produce glucocorticoids and other hormones. These glucocorticoids, cortisol and cortisone in particular, are killers when it comes to thymus cells, a particular brand of thymus cells, killer T cells. Killer T cells are the ones that are primarily concerned with the recognition and destruction of foreign agents in the body including cancer cells. So think positively. And I think my time is up. Thank you very much.

Chapter Eight

WHAT THE FUTURE HOLDS

by

Marilyn Ferguson and Ray Gottlieb, Ph.D.

KRISTIE KNUTSON: It is my pleasure to introduce the next two speakers, Marilyn Ferguson and Dr. Ray Gottlieb. Many of you, I'm sure, are familiar with these two individuals. Mrs. Ferguson is the author of *The Brain Revolution* and of a book which has had a very remarkable effect on many of us, *The Aquarian Conspiracy: Personal and Social Transformation in the 1980s.* Since 1975, she has published an influential international newsletter, Brain/Mind Bulletin. Mrs. Ferguson lectures extensively across the United States, Canada, and Europe, and is, with her husband Dr. Gottlieb, the co-author of a forthcoming book entitled *The Visionary Factor: A Guide to Remembering the Future.*

Dr. Ray Gottlieb received his Optometry Degree from the University of California at Berkeley, and his Doctorate from Saybrook Institute in San Francisco. He is a specialist in vision and learning, and since 1970 he has pioneered training approaches for improving eyesight and visual mental performance in learning and in reading. In 1980 he founded the Eye Gym in Los Angeles. Please join me now in welcoming Marilyn Ferguson and Dr. Ray Gottlieb.

MARILYN FERGUSON: What I would like to do is give just a moment's background to those who don't know *The Aquarian Conspiracy* or the Brain/Mind Bulletin. I assume that probably most of you did pick up copies of Brain/Mind that give you a little bit of a sense of what Ray and I do. We research and publish this newsletter. It has been coming out for eleven years now. *"The Aquarian Conspiracy,"* which was published in 1980, was a description of the phenomenon, that probably everybody here is aware of, which is that there is "something going on." In the midst of all the craziness, in all of the headlines that you wish you didn't have to read, there is something going on that is positive.

That book was my description of the movement that was occurring all over the world, of people who had discovered new realities for themselves, discovered that their own attitudes, the way they looked at life, the way they accepted what happened, and the energy and the commitment they were willing to put out, influenced whether their life was heaven or hell. This may sound like common sense, but you know, human beings have not been long on common sense. It seemed important to say that a lot of people not only had discovered this, but were helping each other to bring a new healing, a new learning, a new way of relating to the world.

Now I was accused of having been overly optimistic and I have to tell you that there were times when I agreed with my accusers. "They're right; forget this transformation stuff; it isn't happening." But Ray and I have been lucky enough and, particularly in the last few years, we have traveled all over the world, and in small towns in the U.S. We've been with top corporate people. We've been with military people and people from basically every category of religion you can think of. In the last few months we've been going from one professional convention to another; we have been talking to people who are highly connected in government, and to people who feel they really represent the most downtrodden. And everywhere there is a leadership that is saying, "Yes, by God, it's happening. The time that we have all dreamed might happen, is happening."

What seems to us that is part of our role, what we need to do in order to make this new paradigm (from the Greek paradigma, meaning pattern), to make this new pattern apparent, is to help show people that it's not unreasonable, that it is logical and scientific, that your left brain can go along for the ride too.

We all know what kind of split we feel if we can't bring our whole self into the picture. David, in one of his psalms, says, "I believe Lord, help Thou my non-belief." And I think we have all felt that. "I know! I'm sure that this is right. I see the light at the end of the tunnel. I'm sure." But there's a part of us that is nervous and doubting. We can't help it. St. Theresa, a great Christian mystic, said, "We may not be able to understand, but it is absolutely important that we try."

The New Age will not be brought in by people who don't want to try to make it logical. There's nothing wrong with logic. Logic is logos, the word, the ordering principle. If we understand enough, we will understand that it all works. St. Augustine said, "Miracles don't occur in contradistinction to nature, but only to what we understand of nature." So we feel that an important thing that we can do now is to talk about vision and that's what our new book is about.

The Visionary Factor: A Guide to Remembering the Future is about the visionary process: how one sees how things might be, and then makes them real, makes them happen. This is a guide for being a practical visionary. We don't want to do this thing fifty years from now, or six generations from now; we want to see it happen in our lifetimes. So there is this kind of delicate tension between patience and will that I think many of you here are familiar with. "I believe Lord, help Thou my non-belief. I want it now, and I will be patient if it can't happen right this minute."

I have to tell you this. Those of you who know me as the publisher of Brain/Mind Bulletin might be surprised to know that I started as a poet and a mystic. I got involved in all this science and brain research because I decided that I wanted to understand the physical side of the mystical experiences that I had. I believe that it's really important that we be willing to bring both our brains together to bring art and science together. As Ray was saying earlier: religion and science. We cannot afford at this point in human history to leave anything out. We have to find how it all fits. Labor and management, Arabs and Jews, Republicans and Democrats—everything, everything has its place in the harmony.

So what we thought we would talk about here today, in the fairly short amount of time that we have (we would like to talk to you for three days), is some of the science. Part of this I would like to contextualize by saying that we're particularly interested in the values to be gained from trying to look at the principles. Instead of just taking fragmented, provocative pieces of scientific break-throughs and letting them sit there as museum pieces, [we want to] see what principles they might indicate to us.

I wish I could remember this word that we made up—it's like you have to bring all kinds of disciplines together. But we made up a word that was something like cyclo-bio-neuro-astro-geo-immunology. Then of course there was pseudo-cyclo-neuro and neo-cyclo-neuro. Albert Szent-Gyorgyi, I think, the two-time Nobel laureate, said one time, "Nature is seamless. Nature doesn't know biology from physics." It all fits together.

We have to be willing to be large enough to let it all fit together and to be willing to be large enough to let all of our multiple personalities co-exist. Within me there can be the accountant, the madcap, and so on and so forth. We try to make ourselves artificially unified, saying, "We've got to get it together." If you notice, we never quite get it together, because we are multiple, we are variable. We are this kaleidoscope of things, just as our sciences are multiple, and just as our religious visions are from our individual eyes, yet they all make one big picture. It's like the "Who I am" can come together when it realizes that it is rich and complex; from that point it becomes more simple.

So part of what we've been looking at is that from the perspective of brain research, new understandings are coming out of the most avant-garde science. There are clues to how some old alternative therapies and insights might have worked, including sound and light. The word light, that is kind of Ray's field . . . so this seems like an appropriate place for Ray to talk about what we're finding now about light and the brain.

RAY GOTTLIEB: . . . Twelve years ago I ran into an optometrist in Oakland who was at the time eighty-one years old. He told me about a therapy called Syntonic Optometry, which had to do with the use of color in a particular device through which you look at a round circle full of color. People would look at it [daily] for twenty-minute periods of time over about two to two-and-one-half weeks. In general it was used for helping children with learning disabilities. The organization, Syntonic Optometry, at this point in time, is about fifty-five years old; we just had our fifty-fifth anniversary meeting. About six years ago I was made the Dean of the College of Syntonic Optometry . . . and what comes to mind is, I remember, as I got into it there were maybe eight people still left in the organization. Most of them were in their sixties and seventies, and most of them are gone now. I came along and influenced other optometrists to get into this. Probably about one hundred or one hundred thirty optometrists are now involved in this area. It has not been easy. . . .

I remember at the beginning, as some of the people from the East Coast, and from the Southwest, and so forth would get together, we had such a strong feeling of history. When we would meet we'd say, "Ah, this felt historic." Essentially . . the therapy . . . [was] for children; it's now expanding. I've used it with a senile lady who had an incredible recovery from it; people have used it with strokes and with certain kinds of other vision pathologies and so forth. It's just now like a rosebud that's about to burst into bloom.

In particular, with learning-disability children, oftentimes you'll find that if you measure the extent of their vision, that is to say, their visual field, instead of having a [normal] visual field, they'll have a visual field that is [restricted]. They have what is called tunnel vision which we all read about, all optometrists and people who are interested in these kinds of things. We heard about hysterical visual-field loss which is this kind of thing, but you never thought you'd ever run into it.

I've done several large school screenings and found that approximately ten percent of children in public schools, or even in private schools, have visual fields that [are restricted]. So you measure this field; you make a determination of which color to use based on their symptoms, based on their history. Do they have a head injury? Do they have allergies? Do they wake up in the morning feeling a certain way? You prescribe a color and they come in and look at the color for twenty-minute periods of time over a period of, as I said, about two-and-one-half weeks.

After about six days the visual field will generally . . . [show improvement], and the blind-spot oftentimes . . . [diminishes in size]. After the two-and-one-half weeks, the eighteen sessions, the visual field . . . and the blind-spot . . . [are dramatically improved]. Along with that goes a change in behavior: more affection, more capacity to learn, willingness to play sports, and so forth and so forth. That was my experience. That was the experience of those of us in this field and yet, the scientific explanation for it was written in the twenties by the man who founded this organization.

To try to get a new paradigm, a new way to look at light, is [difficult because people doubt that] light can affect those kinds of things: light can affect a change in the visual field, light can affect change in the way the brain thinks, or how a person feels. I mean, we're willing to say that this tiny little pill can make me better; that's in our paradigm. But to say that light can do it has been totally dismissed as if it's not a fact, even though I can hold up field charts and say this is what happened, and this is the letter I got from the mother, and this is the one I got from the teacher. It just doesn't exist in the minds—until recently.

Recently there have been several things that have gone on, and one that I'll talk about is a discovery around 1980, 1981, by some psychiatrists who were interested in the field called seasonal affective disorder. I think at the time it was called winter depression. There is, I think, a huge number of people who are suffering from this thing called winter depression, clinically. . . . I think eighty percent of the people who have it, according to one study, never go for treatment. They don't know they're depressed, but their wife or husband or child might know it.

Anyway, what they found out was that if they used large doses, that is to say, bright light for about two or three hour periods during the time of winter when they had these depressions, which would come on generally around November and leave around March, that . . . after a couple of weeks of doing that (sometimes in the morning, sometimes in the evening . . .) the symptoms would go away. And these were people who had been hospitalized and were on drugs. And yet, with that therapy, that non-invasive therapy, [the symptoms] went away.

Recently there was a letter in one of the psychiatric archives that stated that you have to watch it using these bright lights, because you may create something that also exists which makes seasonal affective disorder an even more appropriate term. There is a summer component, flights of mind, where the mind gets really hyperactive. They [also] mentioned possibly spring fever and a kind of summer lethargy as part of this.

Another paper talked about children with learning problems who have their learning problems in the winter time, and nobody notices [the connection]. They are fine, then wintertime comes, they go through this thing, and then in February or March they begin to get better. Maybe it's the pressure of finals, but maybe it's seasonal affective disorder. What they found was that something like seventy-two percent of the adults who have seasonal affective disorder claimed, in one study that they did, that their symptoms started as children. They found eight children, some [of whom were] related to the people who were the other patients, and they did studies where they used light therapy on them. And lo and behold, their learning problems cleared up. A year later when the symptoms came back, it only took a couple of treatments of sitting in front of this light.

Another paper, the one that spoke of the seasonal affective disorder having a summer component and a spring component [indicated] that maybe white light wasn't the best color to use. They suggested in fact, using in the springtime blue-green sunglasses while these people sat in front of these lights, and in the summertime and fall using rose-colored glasses.

In fact, in about three weeks there is going to be a conference in Montreal on Psychophysiology, and one of the main leaders in this field of seasonal affective disorder has a paper in which he is going to describe changes in the EEG patterns on the basis of these children with learning problems having intellectual changes, cognitive capacity increases, and normalization or improvement in what's called visual evoke response, which is a type of EEG problem. So there is a whole field coming from psychiatry that's dovetailing with what we know something about in optometry. I think you'll start seeing that. The Los Angeles Times seems to publish a lot of papers on that; the journal called Science has papers on it, and so forth. I find that very, very exciting.

At the same time there's some information coming out about disease being related to something called free radicals. You might remember from chemistry that sometimes they put these little pluses and minuses next to the carbon, the "C," or the "O" [oxygen] and "plus-plus" or "minus-minus" depending upon what the formula is. If there are too many "plus-pluses" or too many "minus-minuses" running around in your body, then you possibly can have cancer, or then you can possibly have other kinds of diseases. Aging, psychiatric disorders—I mean there's a whole series of things. They're tying the occurrence of many of these kinds of diseases [to] . . . melanin in the body that absorbs this excess of free radicals.

When you have these kinds of diseases, then there is a real increase of melanin which gets shown on the skin, which is related to the uptake of these [free radicals].

A man named Proctor in Houston is writing about that. He sent us three papers recently on it. So there seems to be just now a coming together of information which relates to light, and relates to the fact that in the body there is a light relationship. Perhaps you can even look at the whole physiology of the body in terms of management of light and luminescence. It seems to be coming together now, and it's very exciting.

MARILYN FERGUSON: I was just remembering what our former editor of Brain/Mind Bulletin was telling me yesterday when I told her some of these. This is like the tip of the iceberg. These papers are coming together, and it is just mind-blowing that out of the most remote, highly materialistic measurements of science are coming together these incredible paradigms.

The scientists are so excited and they don't get to talk about it. In other words, they can't put any of that excitement into the [scientific] papers. It's like one of the best-kept secrets around. They feel in many of the sciences now that they are really verging on the break-throughs of the centuries that they have been waiting for.

. . . Some of you may remember the issue we did on melanin about three years ago. Neuro-melanin is related to the melanin that makes the skin dark in sun-tanning, or in racial differences. That melanin is probably the most important molecule for organizing living systems, was the theory of a researcher named Frank Barr from Northern California. He did a paper that was like a huge break-through paper on this theory which got a lot of interest from some Nobel prize-winning scientists and other eminent scientists.

The basic idea is that this very, very black substance may be a major key to understanding mental illness, to understanding the effects of psychedelic drugs, to under-standing aging, cancer, and the ancient mystical idea that man fell from the light and we're climbing back up to the light. And melanin is the thing that is the organizing factor. It is the most sound-absorbent substance known, and the most light-absorbent substance known. It is so black that they couldn't penetrate its structure. It has some mathematical properties that are similar to those of black holes, and it's in all the key parts of the brain. This is really far out stuff.

When our friend Frank Barr was doing this research, they approved it, they published it–these eminent scientists passed off (in terms of their peer review) on this [theory] and nobody quite knows what to do with the information.

We just found out . . . the tests to determine whether a person has been using drugs are not accurate for black people, because the melanin can give the same information as if they were using psychedelic drugs. As I said, "tip of the iceberg."

Ray and I were really excited. We got a paper from a guy in the Department of the Navy—the military can do a lot of outrageous stuff because they're given all kinds of permission to do whatever they want to do—this Navy researcher, and two other people, one from Loyola University in New Orleans, and I can't remember where the other guy is from, had gotten together because they all independently have been working on serendipity, the role of serendipity in science.

Serendipity is such a frivolous sounding thing. What it means, for those who are not familiar with the word, is a happy accident. And what has been coming up is that there are a number of people in science who are now saying, "Wait a minute, the whole history of science is the history of happy accidents. If we don't acknowledge that, we're stifling our discipline." So they did a study. They sent off letters and they said that it was very interesting that Canadian and British science publications (like Nature which is the biggest science magazine in England) tended to publish their request for examples of serendipity in science. The American magazines didn't want to do it.

The American Association for the Advancement of Science, which is the largest scientific organization, did have a one-day symposium a couple of months ago on serendipity in science at their annual meeting. It was heavily attended, against the most strenuous competition at the meeting. The fellow from the Navy who helped organize this said that most of the people who attended were the older and more experienced scientists. He said that the young scientists haven't yet discovered this. They all agreed that what is absolutely the killer in science is that they could not talk about what they really do.

They gave us examples. One reported that he had sent in a paper, and he mentioned in the paper, that the only sample that showed a significant something or other was the one that they had left in the window. The reviewer on the peer review committee wrote back a snide remark and said, "We do not need your meteorological observations." And he said, "They don't realize that that could be important." So they pulled together all of these, [in a] paper that's going to be published in Chemical Engineering, forty examples from all different disciplines [showing] how major scientific breakthroughs have been the results of fortuitous observations, things that were not intended. He said to us on the telephone . . . "Most of the really interesting ones, we didn't have the space to give the backgrounds so people could understand how they happened." But he said, "It begins to appear that this is actually a crisis in science that we have denied that we can talk about how we did it."

Chemical Engineering has been publishing a series of articles that debate on Kekule's Dream. August Kekule was the discoverer of the shape of the benzene molecule. When he was an old man and was being honored at a dinner, he told about how he got it. One time, when he was nodding to sleep before the fire, he was kind of half there, half not there, and all of the sudden, he had this vision . . . of snakes swallowing their own tails. That was what gave him the clue that led him to this discovery, which led in part to the Industrial Revolution.

Now some of the people in science are saying, "He wasn't asleep, it wasn't a dream, and it's very bad for people to think that that's how the creative process works. The creative process works like little bitty step by step by step." So this great debate is going on now in science about Kekule's dream.

Ray got interested in Descartes. He said that Descartes had been misunderstood, and we're blaming everything on the Cartesian duality when that's not what Descartes really meant. But he got his breakthroughs one night, it turns out, in a series of dreams. And these are dreams that he never wrote about, but he told later in his life, and Voltaire recorded.

You see, one of the things that chemists who are down on Kekule's dream said is that he never told it in a scientific paper. We have been all keeping secrets from each other.

One of the things, Ray, that I thought you were going to talk about was the psychiatrist . . . who was using the mirrors. . . .

RAY GOTTLIEB: Someone [a psychiatrist] sent us a paper a month or so ago, and yesterday I got inspired about it and called him up.

In fact it's interesting [to interject here]. Colin Wilson has a new book out. . . called *The Personality Surgeon.* It's about a psychiatrist who discovers, in a series of personal experiences that this one woman. . . when she talked about certain things, her face changed; her mouth changed. That's what the psychiatrist noticed, that whenever this woman started talking about her mother, her face changed. So he said, "Do you have a hand mirror? Just keep it in your lap because I may want to use it." Then she went into that place where she mentioned something about her mother, and she changed her face, her mouth. And he said, "Would you just look at yourself for a second?" She looked and said, "Oh my God, that's the same expression my mother would get on her face when she would do those things to me."

So he [the psychiatrist I called] got more and more involved in this [use of mirrors]. He got involved in saying that maybe there's something to using the mirror in the same way they use Rorschach testing, as a kind of objective thing to look at, that can give you a subjective experience or projected experience. So he began to develop this, and after twenty-five years he's got hours and hours of video tapes of these tremendous kinds of emotional breakthroughs and early life experiences that come to people when he does these mirror techniques on them.

Not long after he discovered the mirror idea, he decided to see what would happen if he used colored light instead of white light. So he began to use colors. I think he said he had seven or eight different colors and it was an accident how he did that one too. Anyway, he said that there are colors that have specific reactions for certain people, almost as if there's an allergy to a color that would bring back an early experience that they had totally [forgotten]. You know how you come up with early experiences that were meaningful, that might have been traumatic for you, and you always had a feeling there might be another one there that you just couldn't remember? Those kinds of experiences, the ones you cannot remember that were significant, would come and the people would be altered from that time on. So there's another serendipity, another approach coming by this man. We'll write about him in the next issue or two of Brain/Mind Bulletin.

MARILYN FERGUSON: We were, the other evening, with our friend Nathaniel Branden who is a psychologist whose work some of you may know. Nathaniel's wife, Devers, has her own approach to doing therapy in which, [as] we found out when Ray mentioned the psychiatrist to her, she does the same thing. She happened upon it totally accidentally herself. Using a mirror, I think even using color, Devers discovered years ago something that the psychiatrist told us yesterday he discovered, which is that the face has two clear sides; one relates to your mother, and one relates to your father. You can tell there are these really remarkable things that can be detected in that way.

These [examples] can't possibly all congeal for you. So please see them as a smorgasbord of examples of the breakthroughs so that you can get your own feelings, because we would like you to feel free to be scientists.

I think it's extremely important that you realize, that we all realize, that the people who created science as we know it today—two to three hundred years ago—were all amateurs. The word amateur means to love. They were so interested, and they were so curious, and they wanted to know, and they didn't have any credentials because there was nobody to give them any. As my former brother-in-law said, "If anybody ever discovers the cure for cancer, he would probably be a dentist." Discoveries tend to be made by people outside the field. People inside the field know too much that's wrong. To be able to have a fresh eye in the mind of a child is really, really important.

There is a new technology that was described in the December 1985 and January 1986 [issues of] Scientific American which is very, very important. Two people we talked to about the time it came out, had said that it was probably going to revolutionize their own field of research. It's called "time-reverse light." Ray will probably have to polish up what I tell you about it, but the simplest description is that a technology was discovered originally by the Russians. The first article in December is by the Russians who did it; they have been collaborating with the Americans. The second article is by one of the Americans, and they are mostly in Southern California.

They use a kind of sandwiching of sound and light waves, pulsed, with mirrors, to create a hologram without film. Is that correct?

RAY GOTTLIEB: It's based on something that is similar to how a rainbow is reflected. A rainbow is reflected by the light coming in, and hitting all these little tiny droplets of water. Because of the arrangement of the water, and because of the refraction of the light, light is reflected out and so you see something that looks like a solid thing out in space. And yet, if you were in the middle of that part of the cloud, or the rain, you wouldn't even know that you were in the middle of a rainbow. So it's a physical non-physical kind of a thing.

The way they produce these phase-conjugate mirrors is as follows: they have what they call a non-linear medium, which is a medium that is responsive to light. It's not inert to light, but actually changes with light. They have this non-linear medium, they have two lasers that come and hit each other this way [gestures], and another laser that comes in this way [gestures] and the two lasers that are coming in this way interact in such a way as to produce sound waves because of their interaction. There is a great relationship between sound and light, acoustic waves, acoustic energy, and photic [light] energy.

So you have these regular light waves coming in creating regular or coherent sound waves. The other light comes in and bounces off these little kinds of particles of sound, these condensed areas, in the same way that light is reflected in a rainbow out of rain drops.

It turns out that the light is reflected by each of these little droplets of sound exactly along the same path that it came on. So that if you shine light through the kind of glass that you have in a shower, or bathroom window, so that it's all dispersed, if that light goes through and hits one of these phase-conjugate mirrors, it gets reflected back exactly on the same path that it came in on, and it hits the piece of glass in exactly the same way, but opposite the way that it came in. It is reconstituted on the other side because it goes through the same distortions, only backwards, and so you can get a strong beam of light coming back. Okay?

The technology provides then a tremendous tool. For instance, one of the tools is this: if you have light reflected from an object and it goes through a lens system, and it hits this phase-conjugate mirror, the light that comes back out, which can be amplified, made stronger, will focus right back on the same target that it came from. So one of the things that you can use this for, for instance, is tracking satellites. A satellite gives off light, the light comes right back exactly the way it came in, and so you can have a satellite up there which is receiving a signal from the earth, and you don't have to focus it. It is focused by itself by using this reflective technique.

What they describe here is that this essentially is a three dimensional, dynamic hologram in space. Holograms have become a real popular way among our kind of folks in thinking about how the brain might work. A hologram is a three-stage process. You have to create it on a photographic plate. You photograph it, you develop the photograph, and then you reconstitute it by bringing back that piece of film with these little squiggly lines on it and put that in the laser light and you get a hologram.

What this allows is a hologram that is created and read simultaneously, because it's created by the light coming in and the light bouncing back from it. So information can come in and interface with information coming in from these [other] two lasers; you can have three pieces of information that come in; and the emergent (the light reflected back out) is a combination of the information, both in terms of space, two dimensional space or three dimensional space, and time. You can code it that way, so that tiny amounts of time or tiny pieces of area can be significant in terms of the tremendous amount of information that it can have.

So you can combine. For instance, in memory you have information coming in, which has to be matched with information stored somewhere in the brain. We have never quite been able to figure out how that works. But in this new technology, the phase-coherent mirror technology, you have a technology that satisfies the requirements for associative memory, for information processing and so forth, that's way beyond anything that we could have even thought of before, except that we knew somehow that the brain needed to have those characteristics in order to be functioning the way we know it. So a few of those people, those scientists, are involved in creating, probably, the Star Wars technology based on this technology, I think.

MARILYN FERGUSON: The Star Wars [comment]—I think that we should clear it up. We don't know that they are using it, but it's the most logical thing and the point I wanted to make about that is the fact that the Russians invented this thing. . . .

RAY GOTTLIEB: The computer of the future will likely be a light computer rather than an electrical computer. The central processing unit will likely be this kind of technology, this phase-coherent mirror. Four-way reflectors is what they call it. Another group of people are interested in applying this to interfacing with how we think that the brain might work. So it's an infant, it's only been around for a few years, but I think that it probably is the discovery of the decade, and will be of tremendous influence on our lives. Also, I think it will help to open up a whole new paradigm and a whole new way of looking at the brain as a light device, an electromagnetic and acoustic device, and will substantiate and further the kinds of therapies and the kinds of healing that we're talking about. . . .

MARILYN FERGUSON: Sound and chanting . . . the healing effects of sound become increasingly reasonable. There's a man whom we met with recently, whose work we're going to write about, a psychologist from Chicago who has a model for healing and therapeutic change that is based on the model of plasma, "the fourth state of matter." He is not saying it is that, but it's like that.

He and various other people, using hypnotic techniques, very sophisticated hypnotic techniques like those of Milton Erickson, are able to create astonishing changes in people. People, for example, who had weight problems can find a way to key into a memory and create another image, and all of a sudden, without real effort they change and they begin to lose weight. The things that used to be thought of as too good to be true, it appears there is reasonable reason why they might be true.

Karl Pribram's holographic model, which many of you are familiar with, I think is going to have a new incarnation in this phase-conjugate technology. It may turn out that the site of the mediation of consciousness is not in the brain, the physical brain, the dense physical brain which is where we have not been able to locate it, as you may know. . . . It may be in fact, that it is in the ventricles of the brain, which are the holes in your head. And we'll probably be doing a Brain/Mind Bulletin on this sometime within the next year where we can piece together all the pieces, so you'll be the first group to hear about it.

Right in the center of your brain there are these interestingly wing-shaped things that look like winged victory (the front part of it) and the ancients believed that this was where the brain dew was and where consciousness was contained. Of course, it all got thrown out. Ray had begun looking at it from the perspective of the optical phase-conjugate mirrors, and we had looked at some other things that were coming out of brain research. It began to look reasonable to think that possibly the processing is occurring in the cerebrospinal fluid in some way, and that the walls of the ventricles, which were originally where the whole nervous system evolved from in the embryo, are the most important site of information.

People have survived incredible brain damage, just incredible! And it turns out that there are hydrocephalics, people with water in the brain, who seem to be quite normal, who have only the thinnest little bit of cortex, the frontal region of the brain which we assumed you have to have to be normal.

So we were saying, "Well, it would seem that if you were shot in the ventricles it should pretty well be fatal." We just got a paper—Ray is really a genius at finding these papers in the scientific literature and sending for them—that says that at least ninety percent of all people who were shot in the ventricles die.

So these, like I said, are just little bits and pieces to say, "Yes light, yes sound, yes psyche, and no, you were not crazy to think that mind is something more than the brain." It's a thrill to me intellectually, emotionally, spiritually, every other way, as this information comes together into such a harmonic picture . . .

What I would like to do is mention . . . just fairly quickly some things that have come up in recent months. One is that heart attacks and strokes tend to cluster at nine o'clock in the morning. (These are things that are coming up in terms of light, timing, things like that, that we would not have known). The brain and the body change sides about every ninety minutes all day long. There's a cross-over period that occurs and the chemistry changes from left, right, left, right, and you breathe out of a different dominant side of the nose, just as the yogis have always said. In fact they have now measured that.

Candace Pert (who is one of the leading scientists in the country and, I think, will win the Nobel Prize one of these days), working with the peptides and the brain opiates . . . recently discovered that the same chemicals that are in the brain are in the immune system, and they ride around on the immune particles in your system. In fact, some of these little particles actually, from time to time, enter the glial cells of the brain, seem to become glial cells, and leave again. It is a zoo! They're finding a zoo of brain chemicals just as the physicists have found a zoo of subatomic particles.

Has anyone seen the show called "Creation of the Universe" on PBS [Public Broadcasting System]? Isn't it wonderful? They were saying, it is so complicated, it is too complicated, and we suspect that what's going to happen is that we're going to find some elegant, simple underlying pattern. There is a feeling of standing on the precipice of that.

Since we're very, very short of time, what I would like to do is to close by reading a couple of things . . . There is a book we saw recently called *Psychobiology of Cancer* in which the author makes the point, reviewed in the next Brain/Mind Bulletin, that boredom may be one of the most important causes of illness. You have an information-processing capability, and if you are not using your optimal processing capability, there's a possibility you will become ill.

In other words, the more you are qualified to do, the more you must challenge yourself to stay healthy. There's another book called *The Psychobiology of Mind/Body Healing* by Ernest Rossi. Rossi is presenting an absolutely luminous model of how our psychic events interface with the body to create illness. I talked to Brendan [O'Regan] last night and I want to give him credit for having absolutely master-minded a whole range of research projects; maybe Willis Harman mentioned them earlier on the mind/body interface.

I think that most of us who are working in this field, almost all of the leading scientists who are working in this field, are artistically and mystically motivated. That's the one thing that they can very seldom talk about, but it's the most important piece of news that we have to somehow get out.

What I want to do is to close by reading three passages from different sources. One from the Desert Fathers reads:

> "Father, according as I am able, I keep my little rule, and my little fast, my prayer, meditation, and contemplative silence. And accordingly as I am able, I strive to cleanse my heart of thoughts. Now what more should I do?" The Elder rose up in reply, and

stretched out his hands to heaven, and his fingers became like ten lamps of fire. He said, "Why not be totally changed into fire?"

The next is just a couple of lines from a song called "The Rose" by Amanda McBroom. Some of you may know it through Bette Midler's rendition of it: "It's the dream afraid of waking that never takes the chance; the heart afraid of breaking, that never learns to dance."

And [finally], this poem [Paracelsus] from Robert Browning, written in the nineteenth century:

> . . . . Thus God dwells in all,
> From life's minute beginnings, up at last
> To man — the consummation of this scheme
> Of being, the completion of this sphere
> Of life: whose attributes had here and there
> Been scattered o'er the visible world before,
> Asking to be combined, dim fragments meant
> To be united in some wondrous whole,
> Imperfect qualities throughout creation,
> Suggesting some one creature yet to make,
> Some point where all those scattered rays should meet
> Convergent in the faculties of man.
> . . . .
> When all the race is perfected alike
> As man, that is; all tended to mankind,
> And, man produced, all has its end thus far:
> But in completed man begins anew
> A tendency to God. Prognostics told
> Man's near approach; so in man's self arise
> August anticipations, symbols, types
> Of a dim splendor ever on before
> In that eternal circle life pursues.
> For men begin to pass their nature's bound,

(in other words we get beyond what it was we thought we were supposed to be)

And find new hopes and cares which fast supplant

Their proper joys and griefs; they grow too great
For narrow creeds of right and wrong, which fade
Before the unmeasured thirst for good: while peace
Rises within them ever more and more.
Such men are even now upon the earth,
Serene amid the half-formed creatures round
. . . .

Thank you.

Chapter Nine

GENERAL DISCUSSION II

with

Marilyn Ferguson, Brendan O'Regan andDrs.
Brauer, Gottlieb, and Wilson

ONSLOW WILSON: Welcome to our final session. I don't know if there are any questions as yet.

MARILYN FERGUSON: This is a question for all of us. . . . A gentleman on the break said that he would be so grateful if we could all come up with a few of our favorite principles that would help tie things together. There is all this information that is very fascinating, but if there [were] a few little statements that you could take away with you, [that would be very helpful]. I love stuff like that. So I am glad he asked. I have a couple, but since I posed the question . . .

ONSLOW WILSON: Go ahead; we don't mind. Ladies first.

MARILYN FERGUSON: The ancient Egyptians called the principles "netters." I don't know if that's the way they pronounced it. . . . Their basic idea was that the way the universe works is that the principles never change, but the circumstances always change. So it's the same old principles but they can be recombined in many different ways given the circumstances. I find that a useful way to think about it. One of my favorite principles was framed by Jose Arguelles, a fellow we know. Some of you may know Jose's works. He wrote *Earth Ascending* and *The Trans-formative Vision.* About a year ago Jose said, "The need for validation is the last obstacle to self-empowerment." If you are going to wait until everybody else tells you it's okay before you can go ahead and do your own thing, you're going to wait a long time. Another friend of ours, Stuart Heller, who lives up in the Bay Area, has eight words, four sentences, that are: "Do nothing"; (basically what that means is . . . slow down, stop) "feel everything; love life; act accordingly." I like tidy little things like that.

This week Ray and I have been working on the *Visionary Factor,* and part of what has happened is that the more deeply we have gotten into it (and we're down to the nitty gritty of putting four years' worth of work together and writing it), the more I realized that people are always saying, this is how the creative person is, and this is how the visionary is. Out here is a description and you should be just like that. You shouldn't be afraid of risking, and so on, but they don't tell you how to do it.

The insights [we have gained from] all the people we have talked to who are really successful at having an idea and making it real in the way they live their lives, all add up to basically this, "If you put as much energy into finding a purpose, and making it happen, as you do in wondering whether you have a purpose, you will succeed beyond your wildest expectations." We spend so much time wondering, second guessing, regretting, and faking it; if [only] we put the energy that we spend in faking it into doing it!

This isn't quite yet into words perfectly, but the basic idea is that, contrary to what you have been told, attraction is very important. What you are attracted to is where your energy is. [Your energy is] not in what you think you should be attracted to. But if you find out what it is that you are being most deeply called toward, that probably is your calling, and if you find some way to make that happen, the chances are you won't be sick.

ONSLOW WILSON: Very true! I have a reincarnation of a question. Apparently the question was asked this morning and we all laughed it away. The person asking the question has not been dissuaded, and so here we are again: "Why was the question on angels not answered this A.M.? Six astronauts saw golden angels while in space. Do you have any comments or observations at all?" We had our comments and observations but obviously they weren't satisfactory so I'll try some more.

ALAN BRAUER: Obviously they weren't there.

ONSLOW WILSON: I visited France this past summer. We spent a few weeks in Paris, working very hard, and one of the things done for me as a diversion, just to get me to relax a bit, was that I was taken to a place called La Géode, which is a spherical theatre. You would sit in this theatre, and you are there. The way they project pictures onto the wall of this spherical theatre, puts you literally in the center of what is happening. I went twice, I was so really taken with it.

The second time I went, I saw a presentation in honor of the astronauts who died on the Challenger, and it was called "The Dream is Still Alive." And I was in space. I knew I was sitting in a theatre, everybody knows that, but the emotion was overwhelming. It really was, sitting there, in a theatre. Imagine then, someone actually being there [in space]. What is going to come up for that person? Imagine them actually being there, and having this experience of the world as one. He or she is in "heaven." Don't forget this is a Christian culture. What will come up for you under those circumstances will be Christian images. This is how I would explain this phenomenon, and they were six Christian astronauts, were they not?

MARILYN FERGUSON: I have met four astronauts and my understanding from them [is that] . . . virtually everyone who has been an astronaut (and I would not be surprised if this were true with cosmonauts), had a transcendental experience of some kind. If you think of us as participatory observers, I think it's possible that the magical, powerful energy of the experience is translated into whatever would be your communication [or conception] of that.

I must confess to you that, one night about three years ago I was sound asleep, and I woke out of a sound sleep and I felt a throbbing or thrumming something that I could only explain to you as angels' wings. It was there for about five minutes—it was incredible . . .

RAY GOTTLIEB: Recently, in the Los Angeles Times, there was a story about the current Pope who, for the last several weeks before that article was written, had been lecturing to his subjects about angels. [He was] talking about hierarchies of angels, and numbers of angels, and their role, and their role in history, and the fact that religion doesn't talk about angels now. I found that fascinating in spite of all the criticism, and the wonder and the uproar that it caused. I never saw an article since then about it, but I thought it was extremely interesting. Also, I find it interesting that the ventricles, those places in the brain we talked about, in some ways look like angels' wings.

MARILYN FERGUSON: They do. After we got interested in the ventricles, we ordered from the North Carolina Biological Supply Company for forty dollars a model of human ventricles. Leonardo [da Vinci] by the way—you remember how he stole bodies so he could study anatomy? One time he poured wax into the ventricles, and scraped everything else away so he could see what they actually looked like; they are winged.

I have a feeling that the reason winged creatures appear, again and again, in our mythology is because we actually have this winged phenomenon inside ourselves, which still doesn't answer your question, because who knows?

ONSLOW WILSON: That's right. All we can do is proffer our particular bias. So you'll have to find your own, I'm afraid.

MEMBER OF THE AUDIENCE: In academia we've been discussing this question for over six hundred years in this form, which is: "How many angels can dance outside a cosmonaut's window?" And we have not reached an answer.

ONSLOW WILSON: I've heard it said, "How many angels can dance on the head of a pin?" Innumerable, obviously. . . .

Okay, I think we can move away from this question at this point. I have a question for Dr. Brauer, and it's a request really. "Please repeat the [name of the] author of the idea that we are 'automatic self-regulating systems' that should not be monkeyed with."

ALAN BRAUER: That's partly a statement that an M.D., Carol McMahon, developed, and also one that I modified, so that's not directly from her work, but my own interpretation and modification of that.

ONSLOW WILSON: This question is not addressed to anyone in particular. I suppose we can all have a crack at it: "How important is exercise and good nutrition in health, or can the mind of itself compensate for the lack of them?" Brendan, do you want to take a crack at this question?

BRENDAN O'REGAN: I think one of the dangers in promoting or attempting to communicate the power of the mind, is to have people go overboard and think that the mind can completely override physical systems. There may be times when dramatic changes can occur, but I think a little common sense would say you've got to keep the physical system in shape.

I think one of the dangers is that when we overdo this role of the mind, we can get into other kinds of problems where people end up being blamed for their illness, and [feel] guilt. Some therapeutic movements have tended in that direction. If you don't get better, they ask, "Why aren't you taking responsibility for your health? Why aren't you getting rid of your tumor? What's the matter with you?" And that's dangerous. So there should be some tempering of this. We have a mind and a body and a spirit and they all have some balance that they need to be in. I would just use the question as a cautionary for that.

ALAN BRAUER: Let me give another angle to that answer . . . that has to do with the importance of exercise in weight loss. There was a study recently completed at Stanford in the Department of Cardiology, Health Improvement Section, to look at the importance of exercise compared with the importance of diet on people who were overweight, because the traditional view is that calories are the most important aspect of weight loss, and that exercise is an ancillary help. But, in fact, what this study showed was the opposite. The group that had exercised only and had no change whatsoever in their caloric intake, had a significantly greater weight loss than the group that had significant calorie restriction and no change in their exercise level. So this certainly says something about the necessity of having exercise just in something as fundamental as weight maintenance.

In my view, there is no substitute for physical exercise. The amount of energy that the brain itself uses is approximately equivalent to half a peanut a day, which is very, very little. And you've got to have that body in motion and not just [be] a piece of dead weight. Remember we're talking about mind and body. The mind affects the body, and equally, the state of the body affects the mind. So you just can't really isolate one from the other. One is not truly a substitute for the other.

ONSLOW WILSON: This one is addressed to "anyone," so the rest of you, out there, can answer it if you have an answer. "What role does the RNA/DNA play in the subconscious healing process?"

MARILYN FERGUSON: I interviewed Ernest Rossi for his book *The Psychobiology of Mind/Body Healing*. He actually describes a mechanism directly from the brain to the RNA as a mechanism of healing. The book was published by W. W. Norton and it's due out this week. . . . It discusses the whole role of RNA and DNA.

ONSLOW WILSON: Two things—we are going to try to have Dr. Ernest Rossi with us next year for our second Annual Metaphysiology Symposium. If we're successful, you'll be the first to know. The second thing I want to say is that it seems to me that there is something that underlies this question, and it is the supposition that the body grows out of RNA and DNA. I'm not so sure that that's what happens. If we accept what Dr. Harman was saying this morning, perhaps RNA and DNA grow out of the mind. Therefore, it is not RNA and DNA that will affect healing, but our mind, and the harmony in our mind, that will affect RNA and DNA. And if what I've heard about Ernest Rossi is correct, this is kind of what he is saying; our profound experiences affect RNA and DNA. It is not the other way around.

MARILYN FERGUSON: There's something about that, too, in the work of Frank Barr, the man who wrote the stuff about melanin. And he has, he thinks, seen a mechanism whereby there is a direct interface . . . an opportunity to actually alter the DNA. It may be right or it may be wrong, but it's certainly exciting.

ONSLOW WILSON: The next question: "I have heard gout likened to male pattern baldness. Are preordained illnesses correctable by inner healing as are traumas and stress-generated illnesses?" I have a problem myself with preordained illness; what do you think, Brendan?

BRENDAN O'REGAN: Well, I was trying to think, as I was realizing what the question was, whether we had any information in our remission data base on remission of diseases that people are genetically predisposed to. Right offhand, I can't answer that, but it's something I'd like to look into. It's something that I can check on.

ONSLOW WILSON: It's interesting that you're likening genetic disorders to preordained illnesses.

BRENDAN O'REGAN: Well, that's a particular form of preordained, anyway, if you want to say that. There is this Dr. Jorge Yunis at the University of Minnesota who is now saying that from a drop of a person's blood he can read the chromosomal mapping in such detail that he can tell exactly at what age someone is going to go bald, for example.

Now, that is potentially dangerous if you think about the health care, health insurance, work, and employment implications of it. That technology, [if it] emerges, [impinges on] the privacy and the rights of the individual. I mean, if you know that someone is going to get cancer at thirty-two (and let's suppose you "know" it with a high statistical accuracy) will you bar that person from educa- tion? Will you educate them properly? What kind of life will they have?

So there are a lot of very tricky questions in this whole notion of what we mean by preordained, but to the extent that that could be reflected, in say, genetically predisposed diseases, I would like to look that up and see. I mean there's Tay-Sachs and sickle cell and there are various other diseases like that, but I don't believe we've had remissions of either of those in our data base. I don't know, I'd have to look for whether there are particular kinds of cancer that are associated with genetic defects in a formal way. . . . We do have remissions of breast cancer, to give an example of a disease that runs in families.

MEMBER OF THE AUDIENCE: Usually there is more than just the one factor. Most illnesses like gout have a genetic component but that doesn't mean that someone with a genetic tendency to manifest gout will actually get gout.

ONSLOW WILSON: Exactly. . . . I am almost wishing that Dr. [Ernest] Rossi were with us today because Dr. Rossi has that really fascinating idea that our deep inner experiences affect our DNA; [they] affect our genes. The reason I am throwing this out again is that I think it is important that you begin to think about [the possibility] that maybe you are not even prisoner to your genes; maybe you do create your own genetic predispositions. . . .

MEMBER OF THE AUDIENCE: Can I ask you one thing? You become aware of things when you become aware of them. . . . If the subconscious mind has such a distinctive decision-making control, what does it take to get a person to become aware of this?

ONSLOW WILSON: If I'm reading your question properly, it seems to me that an adequate answer would be, as the saying goes, "hard knocks and dry falls." When a person gets tired of suffering, then he or she begins to ask questions. That's really how it goes; "Experience is the best teacher" . . . I don't know of any way that anyone has found to force someone else, or to get someone else, to turn inwardly when they are not prepared to do so.

SAME MEMBER OF THE AUDIENCE: But what if you were to show this patient, after thirty minutes, what his body had been doing through his own thoughts?

ONSLOW WILSON: If he didn't want to accept it, he'll find another interpretation. There is a very intimate connection between conscious thought and the subconscious, and, you know, this all has to do with decisions, and it has to do with interpretation, because the business of reasoning, for example, is not at the subconscious level. At least the reasoning that we do, the thinking that we do in our conscious mind, is not at the level of the subconscious. Yet we know that that thinking can have very profound effects at the subconscious level. So there is a very intimate connection, and until the person consciously decides to do something about it, nothing will happen.

Now this [comment from the audience] is real fun: "To all the panel members, after checking *Webster's New World Dictionary,* I learned that the definition of symposium is: 'In ancient Greece, a drinking party at which there was intellectual discussion.'"

I think we are all aware of this definition of symposium, and it seems to me that today eminently qualifies as a symposium, because we have been drinking spiritual nectar.

Here is a question addressed to Marilyn: "How do you feel about the idea of critical mass, and the punctuated evolution theory espoused by Dr. Jonas Salk, which projects instant transmutation of all Homo sapiens simultaneously?"

MARILYN FERGUSON: I don't know what Jonas Salk thinks about punctuated equilibrium, but Stephen Jay Gould and Niles Eldredge are the two people I know who talk about it the most, and they would not agree with that description of what it means. So I think we've got about three different theories a little mixed in together there. Punctuated equilibrium is an idea that evolution occurred very intensely at certain times, in certain species, possibly due to the stress of circumstances. . . . Very rapid mutations seem to occur when a species is at the end of its rope, so to speak, at the edge of a terrain that it has been familiar with, or where the climatic circumstances suddenly change.

This suggests the possibility that evolution occurs because of necessity, and that we're driven by the need to evolve.   This fits in nicely with the work of Ilya

Prigogine, who won the Nobel Prize in 1977 for something called the Theory of Dissipated Structures, which is basically that in living systems, when the energy level gets to a certain place, the old structure can't handle it any more and it falls apart and then reorganizes itself at a higher level of complexity.

There is definitely evidence, although nobody can figure out why, for some kind of an attraction in evolution, something that keeps moving us ever onward and upward. There's a whole field of mathematics called dynamic chaos (and it's got some other names), and it refers to what they call "strange attractors" which I think is such a cute expression. We've all met strange attractors. . . . The strange attractors are mathematical models that can be tracked and seem to drive things into a certain shape. Nobody knows how or why.

Let's face it, we don't understand how aspirin works. If you look up fire in the encyclopedia you'll find that they quote poets, because nobody knows [what it is]. The fact that water occurs was not to have been predicted—not that we were around to do the predicting! We really need to face up to the fact that there are mysteries that we are better off describing than trying to explain.

RAY GOTTLIEB: I think history works in the same way. We have bursts of history, bursts of historic spirit that come' out, and the talk about evolution reminded me of the kind of experience which for me was important. It was realizing that by applying ourselves to the development of the kind of things that we're talking about here today in terms of self-healing, and by applying ourselves as a society, and as individuals, and as a world, to the development of the use of our own intelligence, [we can] develop an even greater intelligence. That idea hit me so strongly one day that I think I was altered, that I evolved in that moment. We can decide to evolve ourselves through developing our intelligence and our powers. I think the time of that is here, and I think that's apparent.

MARILYN FERGUSON: In fact, Ray came up with a metaphor that I thought was really neat. Just as at one time in a long distant past, our ancestors, who were hunters and gatherers, discovered agriculture (they didn't have to wait for the accidents of the harvest and so on, but they did actually make it happen), we may be right now discovering the cultivation of intelligence. This is not a static thing. Intelligence can be trained. Adults can continue to evolve their intelligence. The synapses, the connections between the [cells of the] brain, are plastic and continue to change. If this is true, if this is right, then this is probably one of the most significant times in the history of the human species.

ONSLOW WILSON: I would like to add, apropos of evolution, that you, Marilyn, started this whole thing off with the business of principles . . . so I would like to get to the principle of evolution. If there is such a thing as a principle of evolution, then clearly the hallmarks will be recognizable. And I think that anyone who is involved in self-transformation will know how evolution works, because if it's a principle, it will manifest within us as individuals, it will manifest in the society as a whole, it will manifest in species, it will manifest in galaxies, etc. We really don't have to go any further than ourselves to discover the principle of evolution and how it actually unfolds.

MARILYN FERGUSON: What I like is the way the principles kind of knit together. . . . We seem to know now that we tend to evolve through stress and challenge; if you're suffering, you start to ask questions. We can get smart, and start doing what we need to do before the pressure gets too hard. We could volunteer to change and, in fact, I think that is what has happened to a lot of people, and that is why the people who are here [at this Symposium], are here. That is a better way than waiting until the screws are tightened [to force] you to bring about the changes you need.

ONSLOW WILSON: The next question is: "Would you comment on the ability of children to quickly overcome most illnesses and to adapt in a positive manner to what seems to be catastrophic diseases?" Who wants to grab that one? Brendan, you talked a lot about diseases and stuff in the immune system.

BRENDAN O'REGAN: Well, we have noticed that in the reports on remission so far, [remissions] tend to [be] happening either in the very young, or, curiously, in the old. They don't tend to be happening in the thirties and forties. It's at either end of the spectrum. In some cases I suppose, you would say that may be not surprising, that it would happen in the young. But in some ways it is, because their immune systems are not fully formed.

For example, one of the problems that happens in young people getting transplants (kidney transplants and so forth) is that, because their immune systems apparently aren't fully developed, when exposed to Epstein-Barr virus they come down with lympho-proliferative disease. And so in some sense they are more vulnerable, but in certain other kinds of conditions they do seem to be able to go into remission. For instance, children will frequently go into remission from neuroblastoma.

We had a call recently from a woman, who had a child who had a particular kind of heart problem, and wondered if there was any evidence of remission of that, and we found eight different reports of remission and shipped the papers off to her. The doctors looked at them and said, "Where did you find this?" They were a little bit surprised. On the basis of reading the papers, [they] decided not to put the child through surgery and to wait to see if it would resolve naturally. And it did. So the child was spared the trauma of surgery.

ONSLOW WILSON: Here's a question for Dr. Brauer: "Can AIDS be a phenomenon of epidemic hysteria, which is a precursor of the, or of a, paradigm shift, which is being manifest on a biophysical level?"

ALAN BRAUER: Epidemic hysteria reminded me of an interview question that a reporter from Peninsula Times posed to me several weeks ago. I don't know if any of you have read about the infestation of the garlic-smell poison case. . . . Well, there were some mysterious shipments that arrived in a number of different offices in the Bay Area that smelled a lot like garlic. A garlic smell is characteristic of a very serious kind of poison.

So authorities were concerned that some mad poisoner was shipping these to poison a number of different offices. A whole lot of people started getting seriously ill, and were taken to the hospital with this case of poisoning. It turned out, as they investigated the source of this, that this garlic-like smell was garlic, and everyone got well right away. Now that's a case of epidemic hysteria.

I wish that AIDS were as simply treated. But the fact is that AIDS is a virus that has indeed been isolated, and it is not the figment of anybody's imagination. Who gets it, though, is a lot more variable, and this conforms to the usual laws of epidemiology. Even a virulent kind of a virus, or bacteria, is not going to create an illness in every single person who has it in their systems. That has to do with all kinds of complex issues of immunity. So obviously, you want to do whatever you can to keep your immunity at the highest, and certainly try to avoid getting infected, if possible.

This is why the information is being put out about the known methods of transmission, so that people can make intelligent choices in preventing exposure, and that's the way to prevent the spread until a vaccine is found. Even if there is not one found, that doesn't mean that everybody is going to get it and die—definitely not! It just means that there is going to be a certain increasing percentage of people who will become infected.

Even [among] those who become infected and contract the disease, not every single person ends up with death. This is still another factor in the immunity response, and if your immune system is weak, but not that weak, you may recover. So you need to do whatever you can to keep your immune response as strong as possible, and try to avoid getting infected. Know your partners!

ONSLOW WILSON: You see, microbes, viruses, and so-called disease-causing agents have just as much right to be here as we do. So the attempt to annihilate them is kind of futile. What we really need to be doing is learning how to control our own emotional reactions and, therefore, keeping our immune system in the best possible fighting shape. That's basically the challenge, not trying to annihilate viruses, and bacteria, and so on. These are nature's children, just as we are.

DONNA BRAUER [wife of Dr. Brauer]: I'm reminded of a young man who not only had AIDS but had herpes; his parents brought him in because he was in very bad condition. He came in very stressed, and very depressed, and said he was going to die. Well, Alan and I worked with him, and we convinced him that he didn't have to die. In fact, he could take this as a challenge. And not only could he take it as a challenge, but he could break some of the records of some of the people who had AIDS; he could succeed where others had failed. We gave him the challenge of living for five years. Well, we taught him relaxation exercises, and his herpes got better; he stopped taking the eight or nine codeines per day for his pain; he was improving dramatically and he was at home with his parents. He got so well that he decided to move back to his former environment. Well, we strongly advised him not to do that, because he was doing so well. Unfortunately, he did. And he died.

We felt very strongly that when he was working in a positive environment, when he was in a different environment that was a healthy environment, when he had a challenge and a support system, that his entire health had changed. His body was changing. He was hopeful. He was encouraged, we were encouraged, and that made a difference. Unfortunately, he lost that.

MARILYN FERGUSON: My brother died of AIDS about a year ago . . . and he had actually had two, or three, miraculous remissions, and the same thing happened that you're describing. I said to him, "It's your consciousness, you're not over it, you have to maintain that consciousness." He got too much chutzpah! It was in the same matrix, the same downward spiraling psychological pattern. And he realized that, but he realized it too late. So I absolutely agree. I saw miracles happen with him, so I know that it can go either way. I do not know how long it might have lasted, but I saw the same thing you describe.

ONSLOW WILSON: This one is addressed to you, Brendan: "Could you please talk a little more about schizophrenia as viewed from a virus immune system viewpoint? Also, how could one provide hope for the mentally ill? It would seem the helpless outlook now held would certainly depress the immune system."

BRENDAN O'REGAN: There's a paper by Candace Pert on the idea of schizophrenia as an auto-immune disease, which was published the latter part of last year. Again, it's something [for which] I have the reference, but not in my head, but if whoever's asking [would] send me a card reminding me that you want that (with your name and address), I'll send you that paper. There is definitely a move afoot to think that neuropeptides research will yield some treatments here by blocking certain neurotransmitter production also affecting the receptor sites in the nervous system. Glaxo Corporation, which is the biggest British international drug company, has in testing stages now, a neuropeptide treatment that they believe will help schizophrenia. That happens to quite independently fit in with

Candace Pert's hypothesis.   So there is some sense there that something can be done.

These are all substances that are not like the major drugs that we use and think of now. They appear to be rather simple strings of amino acids that may be anywhere from five to eight or fifteen amino acids long.   And they're basically looking at what kind of structure they fold up into (the secondary and tertiary structure of them when they're in vivo) to see what kinds of geometry they must have to fit in these receptor sites.

This is a little on the speculative side, but it is at the trial stage with Glaxo. Candace has done [research] with peptide T and other analogues of that at NIMH [National Institute of Mental Health]. (If they just would get around to testing some of these things they may reach us sometime soon. There has been a viral notion about schizophrenia for some time, but no one has known what virus and where it would attack.) Her notion—I'm just passing on an opinion—is that it may attack the same receptor sites on the T cells or receptor sites related to the ones that she's been studying. And if you want detail on this, let me know who you are and I'll send you the reference.

ONSLOW WILSON: This question is for both Marilyn and Alan, but somehow it says: "Marilyn, you mentioned that negative memories buried in the subconscious mind can be changed and brought into the conscious mind by a special method, such as used by Erickson, of reprogramming. Isn't this what a hypnotherapist does? Please elaborate."

MARILYN FERGUSON: Basically, that is what hypnotherapists do, and I think that the thing I'm interested in is that some of them have very, very effective . . . experimental techniques.   Rossi does, this fellow Bill Cheshire from Chicago does, and there are many others, and many therapists who use things that are similar to hypnotherapy who are able to catalyze powerful change.

The complimentary [issue of] Brain/Mind Bulletin called the "The New Models of Imagination, something-something" [tells about] a psychiatrist who actually uses what he calls "imaginal thinking," not specifically to unlock memories, but to provide a very powerful visual image of healing that he has used with a number of patients having a number of different illnesses.

The point that he makes is that the imagination is real; the realm of the imagination is real. It transcends time and space; it does not have limits. The reason it can effect healing is because . . . it has no past and it has no future; it's just there to be used and it is qualitatively different. We could spend the whole day on how that might work. The most important thing is that it is effective, you can see it work. People should be very careful of what they are doing when they start fooling around with hypnosis because it works well enough that . . . if you don't know what you're doing, you can actually establish some things in people that might be negative or a little bit off. . . . It really does work, so you should be careful of it.

ALAN BRAUER: Well, I see hypnosis as simply an altered state of consciousness where a person is more suggestible to outside influences, and also more aware of interior influences, of the subconscious. I'm a little less worried than Marilyn is about the dangers involved. Our basic regulatory control mechanisms are not going to allow us to do things that are dangerous for us, or against our beliefs.

Anything that is programmed during a hypnotic or trance state is not likely, in any one session, or even several sessions, to be lifetime permanent. In fact, that is one of the reasons that hypnosis is not as ultimately powerful as we would like it to be, because it doesn't have such a permanent effect. It has to be reinforced by one's own self-hypnotic abilities. So you have to be very much in agreement with any kind of suggestion coming in for it to have a really permanent effect.

[Discussing] how to get to the unconscious, could occupy a great amount of time. Essentially, what you want to do is get the conscious mind quiet, and listen, and look, and feel. What comes up is coming from your subconscious. But if you are too busy looking outside, and listening to all the noise from your conscious [mind], or from the exterior environment, you are not going to hear what is happening inside. So anything that you can do to quiet your conscious mind is going to allow you, if your interior senses are ready, to look, listen, and feel.

RAY GOTTLIEB: I think it might be fruitful for me to describe one session that I saw Bill Cheshire do and I'll try to give you the principles of it. Essentially, what he believes is that we live by a series of stories. We carry those stories in us. Those are images which are in a story form. He feels that if you can change the story, if you can create a new story, that in one session you can change a person's life, because they don't look at [the old story] any more; they don't have the same patterns that they are going to keep using.

Essentially the way he does it, from my perspective (and I have to say that if he were here, he may have his own way of saying it, or maybe that I'm saying something that's not quite right) goes like this. He listens for awhile to the person [the patient], interviews them, and then gets a sense of where the story might be. Because he knows so many different people from his own experience, he can feel that the story is there. Then what he does is he takes the person back in terms of their own experience, from their own interview. He uses words like "the sidewalk that had bricks in it" or "holding my father's hand with this hand," details [from the patient's own interview].

So he gets the person into that past experience, and then he gets them confused. He feels that in the state of confusion, the mind is open to re-formation, to reforming the story. By confusing, I'm not talking about something huge, or dangerous. [For instance], he asked the person that I saw, "Was it your left hand that your father held, or your right hand?" And you could see her going through the question, trying to get inside, and saying, "Well, maybe it was on my left side, maybe it was my right side", and he stayed with that very patiently—a lot of time between words, a lot of space. Then he said, "Well, let me take you through an experience."

He took her [the patient] into an experience by having her in the story of a little girl who had a rabbit, which was symbolic, and also represented something to her that he had seen her react to. . . . [He said], "Look at that beautiful little rabbit, it's so soft." He knew that she had this emotional attachment to that [rabbit]. Then he said, "The child then goes in and takes a nap." And, "goes in and takes a nap," was the [hypnotic] induction.

So she's having this story told to her, and in her dreams she dreams something about her experience with the rabbit. In the dream, the girl goes and takes a nap, and has a vision about the rabbit. Then she wakes up from the nap, the story ends, and she comes back to being where we were. So that's a description.

But the principle that seems to be very important (and there seem to be a couple of principles there) is the idea that in the state of question, in the state of where you have to be open to find the answer, there's a physiological change. The physiological change has to do with long-term and short-term memory, the RNA factor. And in that state [of question], you can recreate the story, by using bits and pieces, that then can change the person's life because the story has changed.

MARILYN FERGUSON: The rabbit story that he made up—and, by the way, he practices on his children; he tells his little girl stories every night before she goes to bed;

she won't let him off the hook—was a beautiful [story] like a positive fairy tale, a comforting kind of image.   He believes he is, in effect, creating a whole new hologram.

ONSLOW WILSON: It sounds to me that what's happening here is a sort of re-interpretation of an experience. This is something that I think is very, very important; it is something that we, as Rosicrucians, stress.   You can go back to past experiences that have been traumatic, and you can re-interpret them, but you must have that willingness, that disorientation, that openness, that questioning.   It's a time when you will have an insight as to how best to re-interpret this situation. It releases you from it.   And yes, the story is changed.   The elements are still there but they're changed; their relationship has changed.

RAY GOTTLIEB: In the experience something came up that was very important.   As we watched him [Bill Cheshire], the emotion that he felt was almost identical to the emotion that she [the patient] felt at the same time. So we talked about that.   He talked about [the fact] that when he was telling the story, which made itself up as he went along, he had his eyes closed, and so did she.   He said, "It was as if we were in a room together, and I had a slide projector.   I would project the slide of the next part of the story."   He started out with a squirrel in the story and then he changed it to a rabbit.   He said, "What happened was that I looked, and I could see the emotional reaction of the woman I was working with inside this little theater." . . .   In fact, before he said what the next part of story was, the slide of the image of it would flash up in his mind, he would feel her reaction to the slide, and vary his story according to her reaction, even before he said it.

ONSLOW WILSON: That's attunement.

MEMBER OF THE AUDIENCE: Has he worked with patients with schizophrenia?

MARILYN FERGUSON: I think he works with a lot of people.   He specializes in people with obesity problems.

One was a woman who worked for me at the time, and she was leaving my employ, but he was coming up to see us, to demonstrate what he did, be interviewed, and to help with some brainstorming. So I had asked her if she would like to pick him up from the airport, and drive him up to Lake Arrowhead, which is where the meeting was. He ended up putting in about three days with her. She told me, the last time I talked to her, that she had lost, in a little over two-and-one-half weeks, fourteen pounds. . . . In most approaches to obesity, about two percent of the people keep the weight off over [a period of] two years. But of the patients that he followed up, something like twenty-five percent have kept, or increased, the weight loss, and they all did it with no particular effort.

RAY GOTTLIEB: I want to say something that I read in Ernest Rossi's book, who also happened to be the other person with us watching Bill Cheshire do his work. What he said was that one of the early people . . . who wrote about hypnosis made a statement that hypnosis is the state of "no doubt." The idea becomes vision, or becomes completed, before that part of your mind that doubts can come in. So somehow, it is a quieting down of that part of your mind that doubts and squelches the imagery. . . .

I thought that sense of "no doubt" (if you expand that), really talks about a lot of things that we learn about, and study about, and that come across in [Dr. Brauer's presentation]. Another piece of information that occurs to me is that there are people who are highly hypnotizable, and there are people who are not very hypnotizable, it seems. It turns out that charismatic leaders are people who are extremely hypnotizable. What occurred to me was that a charismatic leader leads from a place of "no doubt," and if the audience or the followers are going into the field of "no doubt," they follow.

ONSLOW WILSON: You're speaking of what we call attunement.

MEMBER OF THE AUDIENCE: Dr. Brauer, as a logical extension of walking on fire, shouldn't one also be able to walk on water?

ALAN BRAUER: That comes in next year's Symposium.

MARILYN FERGUSON: How many of you have seen the movie "Being There," with Peter Sellers? Remember at the end of the movie what happened, as he walked out on the ice which was like the equivalent of walking on water.

ONSLOW WILSON: Isn't there a story of a Chinese Buddhist who got so involved with his meditation that he started walking? He was walking beside a lake, and suddenly, he was walking on water, and then he lost his concentration, sank, and drowned.

MEMBER OF THE AUDIENCE: What research is being done with sound effects, specifically verbal sounds and intonations?

RAY GOTTLIEB: First of all, there is a new sound technology, called holophonic sound. The difference between monophonic sound and stereophonic sound, if you're sensitive, is great. The difference between stereophonic sound and holophonic sound is out of this world. [To illustrate] you are hearing me now sitting here in front of you in a specific location with respect to you; and you can hear the three dimensionality, you can hear the other people coughing, and moving around, and so forth. If there were a plane, you would hear a plane overhead.

On a normal stereo, you won't hear it that way, [although] you will hear something. On a holophonic sound, it is as if you are in the location, specifically, where the sound is located. It is just as if you were closing your eyes and hearing it now. Most people don't realize that when we hear stereo, we're not hearing as if we were there. This [holophonic sound] is 360-degree, spherical sound, located in space. It's amazing! It's eerie! So that's one thing that is happening, and I think the application of that both to healing, and to education, will be quite profound in the next few decades.

There are other things going on. There is a type of binaural presentation. In wave-vibration applications, there's something called beats. If you take a tuning fork, and [another] one that's slightly off, and you hit both of them, you'll not only hear the tone, but you'll hear beats. What they've done is put various frequencies of sound, say 400 cycles a second, in one ear, and in the other [ear] 405 cycles a second. So you get a beat of five cycles a second because that's the way the two frequencies mesh.

They feel (and I think they've done some measurements on this) that they are influencing brain-wave patterns. So, if they wanted to have someone, say at an eight-cycle-a-second brain wave pattern, they could produce it, or have the person move into it, by having this binaural presentation with the beats. They claim that they used it in a school room, where they had it (but not on ear phones) constantly going, with the sound of music, or waterfalls, in the background, kind of masking it a little bit. According to their report, which was not a scientific report, but a description and a testimonial, there was a great change in the capacity of the children to learn, to not be stressed, and to have greater self-confidence. I think the Monroe Institute calls this technique "Hemispheric Synchronization."

So there seem to be some things that we will receive the fruits of in the next years. I think that the coming together of light and sound in technology is there. We have crossed the bridge for that, and I think that we will begin to understand that relationship, and the importance of that relationship, for our own functioning and our well-being.

MARILYN FERGUSON: We got impatient waiting for someone to produce a holophonic tape, so we got together with the inventor, and did the sound effects, and some symphonic music. It's listed inside . . . that [Brain/Mind]

Bulletin if anyone is interested. I noticed that the jet plane on there [the holophonic tapes] is very powerful. We think of that [the sound of a jet plane] as a negative experience, but if you allow those jet engines to go through your body, it can be very positive. . . . I think we're just scratching the surface.

ONSLOW WILSON: The Nigerians, at the University of Ife, are also working a lot on this, on chants, and so on. You may be interested in this.

On this note I think our discussion is over. I think our emcee has a few words to say to you. I want to thank you personally for being here. It's been a wonderful day. The negotiations went well; we got good weather. The food was good I'm told. Thank you.

CLOSING REMARKS

KRISTIE KNUTSON: You know, many years ago, Tutankhamen's tomb was discovered, and after great effort they managed to get a hole into the interior of the tomb. Howard Carter was given the privilege of being the first to look inside. He put a candle inside, stuck his head in, looked, and was totally silent. The others around him were saying, "What do you see? What do you see?" They were so curious! After a moment, because he was so dazzled by the beauty and the glory of what he saw, all that he could whisper in awe was "wonderful things."

As we, today and tomorrow, continue this process of unfolding life to ourselves, unfolding ourselves to ourselves, and unfolding the creative principle of God to ourselves, how can we help but perceive the dazzling, glorious beauty of that? How can we help but whisper to ourselves, in awe and gratitude, and whisper to each other a great, growing, cleansing, healing whisper flowing across the face of this earth—"Wonderful things, my God, wonderful things".

Thank you for being with us today.